The Funny Side Collection

The Fart Side
Blowing in the Wind!

(Pocket Rocket Edition!)

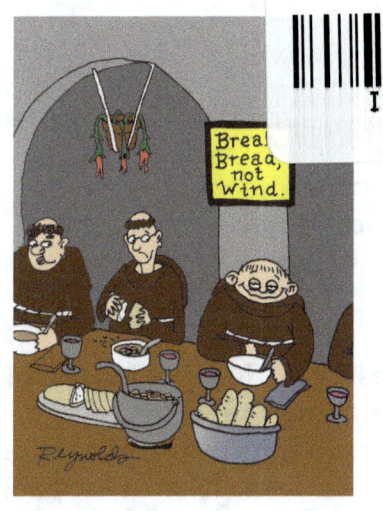

Dan Reynolds
Joseph Weiss, MD

© 2017 Dan Reynolds
Joseph Weiss, M.D.
SmartAsk Books
Rancho Santa Fe, California, USA
www.smartaskbooks.com

All rights reserved. No part of this book may be reproduced, reused, republished, or retransmitted in any form, or stored in a database or retrieval system, without written permission of the publisher.

ISBN-13: 978-1-943760-13-8 (Color Pocket Rocket)
ISBN-13: 978-1-943760-36-7 (e-Book Pocket Rocket)
ISBN-13: 978-1-943760-58-9 (Color Print Expanded)
ISBN-13: 978-1-943760-63-3 (e-Book Expanded)

The Fart Side: Blowing in the Wind!

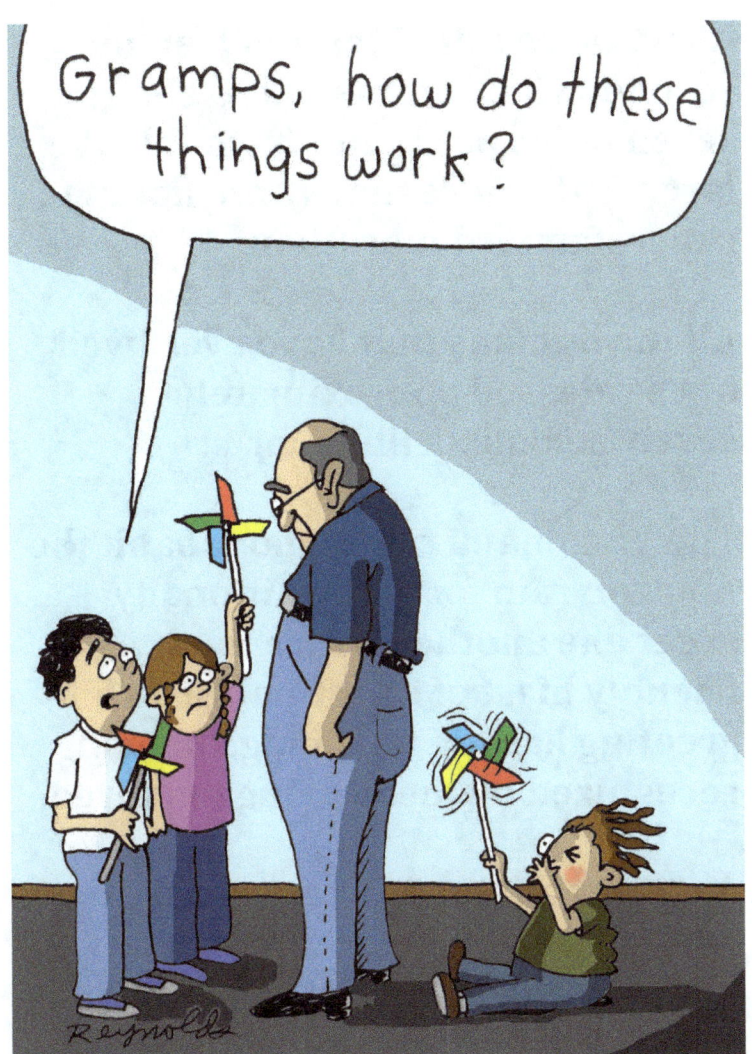

The Funny Side Collection

A fart travels at about ten feet per second, which works out to about seven miles per hour. It would take a fart a little more than three hours to run a standard marathon.

All the humans that have ever lived have released approximately seventeen quadrillion farts.

The Yanomami tribe who inhabit the Amazon rain forest traditionally greet one another with a loud, friendly blast of intestinal gas. The greeting has the advantage of being recognized by the hearing impaired.

A tighter anal sphincter gives rise to a louder fart. If you fart loudly you can take some pride in the fact that your anal sphincter tone is in good form.

The Fart Side: Blowing in the Wind!

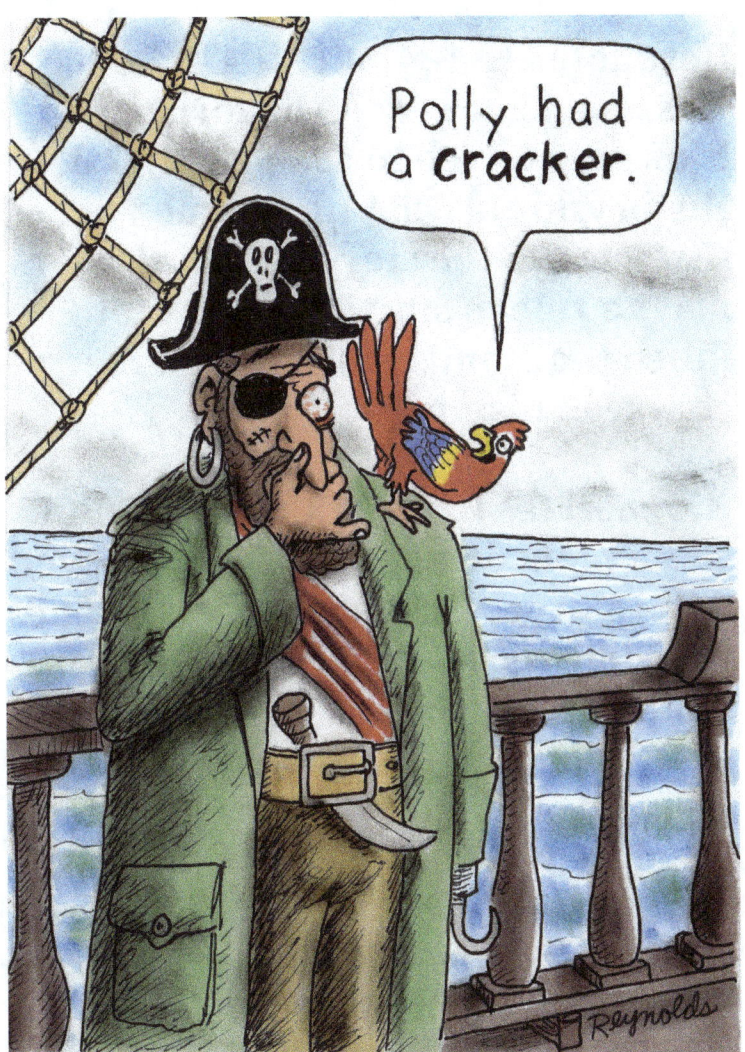

The Funny Side Collection

Herodotus (c.484 BCE – c425 BCE) was an ancient Greek historian, and is often referred to as the Father of History, for his classic volume *The Histories*. In the story of Apries, a fart plays a role in starting a war that killed thousands and changed the course of history.

Hippocrates (c. 460 BCE – c. 375 BCE) was a pioneering physician who lived during Greece's Classical period, and is widely recognized as the father of modern medicine. As early as 420 B.C. Hippocrates had warned of the dangers of holding in a fart, as he wisely wrote in *Treatise on the Flatuosities*: "It is better for it to pass with noise, than to be intercepted and accumulated internally".

The Fart Side: Blowing in the Wind!

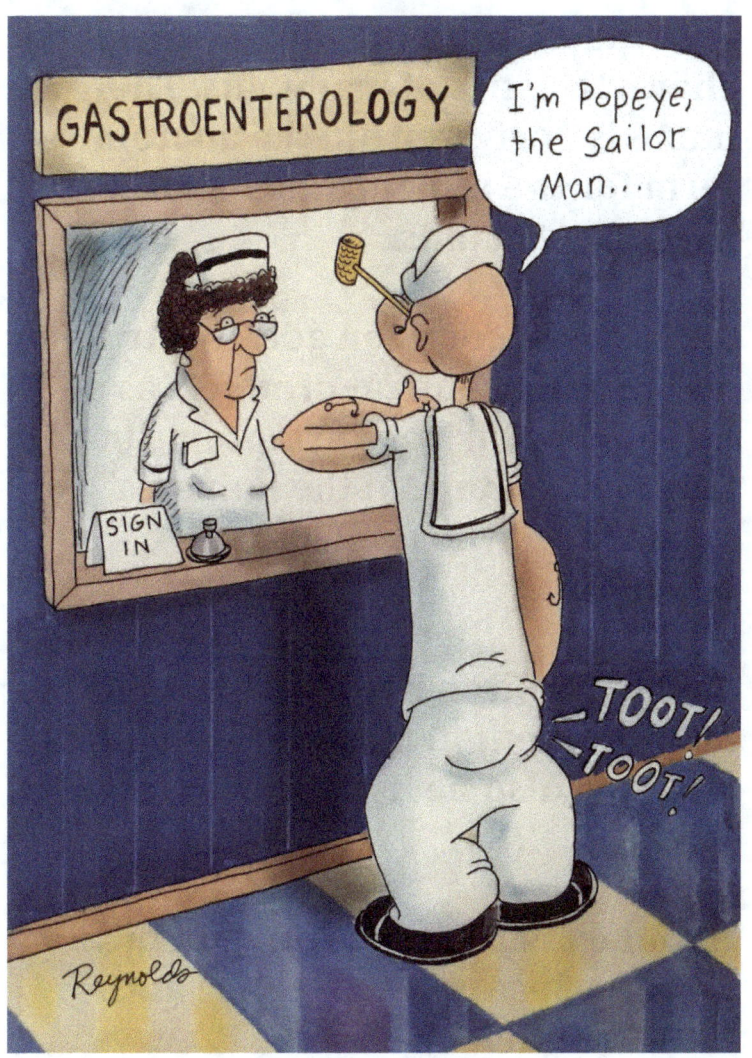

The Funny Side Collection

Feeding their young milk is one of the characteristics of mammals. Their name is derived from the anatomical term for the milk producing breast, mammary glands.

Lactose is a common additive to foods and pharmaceutical products as a filler. It may trigger symptoms in the large percentage of the human population who are lactose intolerant.

Lactose is often not clearly labeled as an ingredient in foods and products, and may also be listed as nonfat dried milk.

Hypolactasia is the formal medical term for lactose intolerance and lactase deficiency.

The Fart Side: Blowing in the Wind!

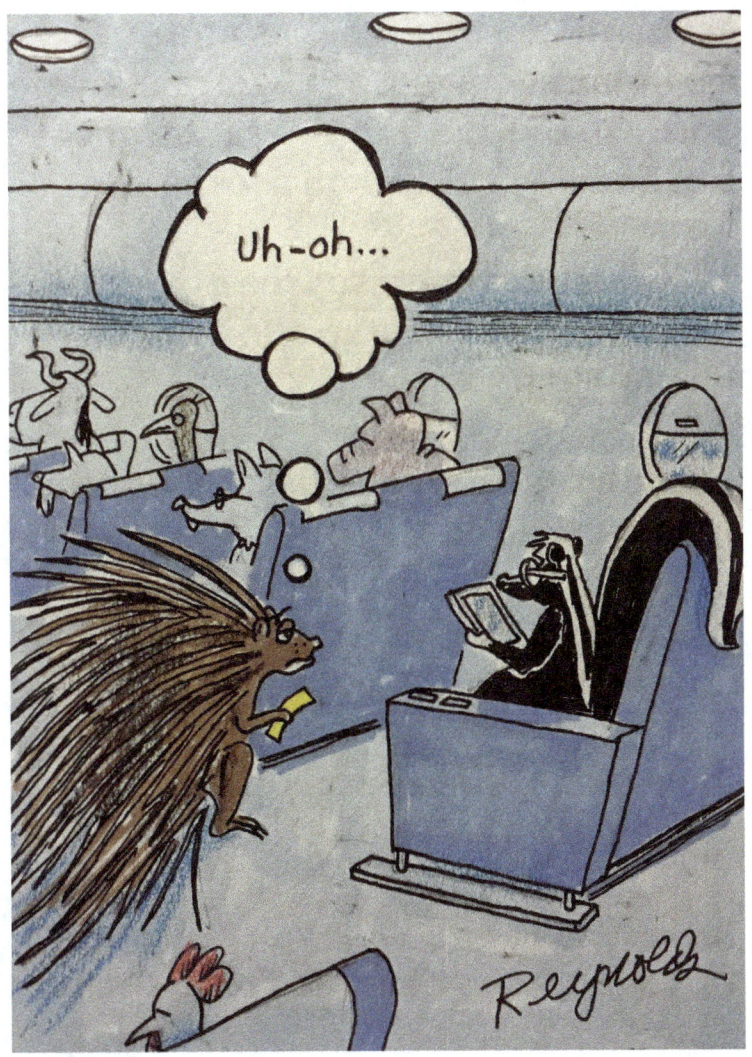

The Funny Side Collection

Scuba divers avoid beans and carbonated beverages before a dive because the gas bubbles in the gut can become painful on ascent.

The most common source of intestinal gas is air swallowing (aerophagia).

The average person passes more than ten farts per day.

The aroma of a fart can be an indicator of intestinal health.

Over ninety-nine percent of the gas passed in a fart is odorless

Ice cream is often forty percent air by volume, and contributes to intestinal gas.

The Fart Side: Blowing in the Wind!

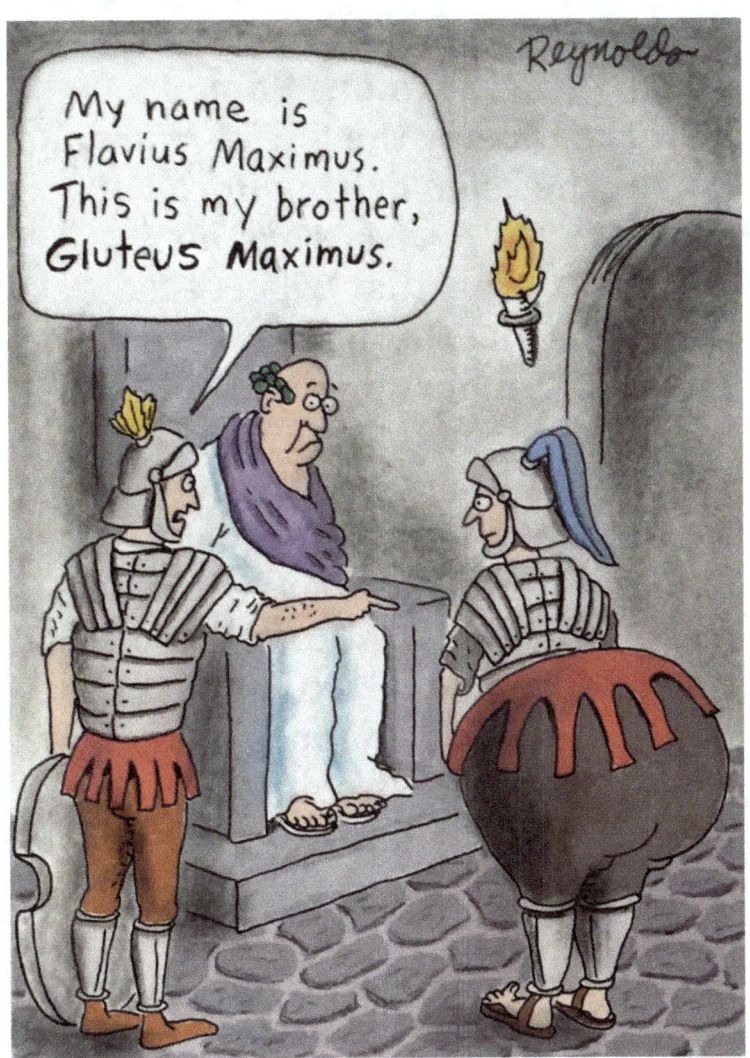

The Funny Side Collection

Titus Flavius Josephus (c. 37 AD – c. 100 AD) was a famous Roman historian during the Jewish Wars and during the reign of King Herod of Judea. In *The Jewish Wars*, he describes a fart that triggered a stampede and the deaths of twenty thousand innocent people.

Saint Jerome (Latin: Eusebius Sophronius Hieronymus (c. 347 AD – 420 AD) church scholar, historian, translator, and prolific writer offered the following admonition: "It is good neither to eat flesh nor to drink wine – but with beans also anything that creates wind or lies heavy on the stomach should be rejected. I think that nothing so inflames the body and titillates the genitals as undigested food."

The Fart Side: Blowing in the Wind!

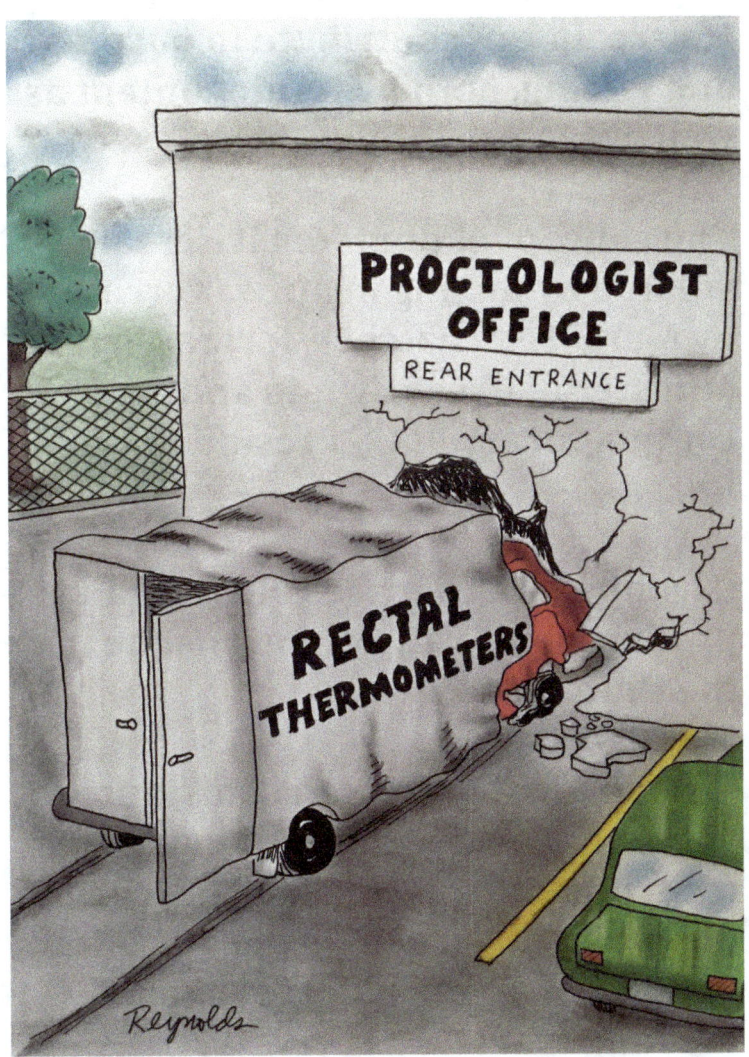

The Funny Side Collection

Ice cream can contribute to burping and farting, both by its air content as well as lactose intolerance.

The concept of doubling ice cream volume by mixing in air was created by Margaret Thatcher, former Prime Minister of Great Britain and a contemporary of US President Ronald Reagan.

Carbonated beverages outsell dairy products by a ratio of four to one in the United States.

Carbon dioxide gas can contribute to burping and belching. It does not contribute to farting since the carbon dioxide is absorbed by the gut, enters the bloodstream, and is exhaled by the lungs.

The Fart Side: Blowing in the Wind!

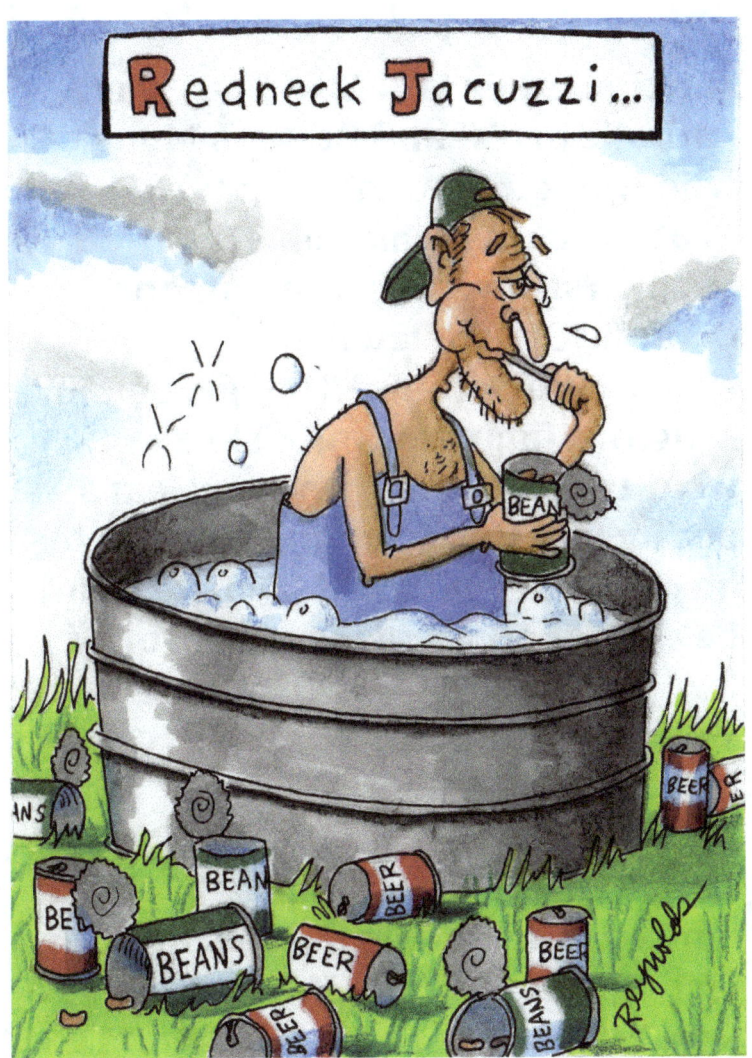

The Funny Side Collection

Martin Luther (1483 – 1546) was a Catholic priest and German Monk who was a major figure in the Protestant Reformation. His confrontations with the Roman Catholic Church led to his excommunication. Although a major religious figure his published writings and letters embrace earthy bodily functions. Farting appears to be one of his personal favorites, and he described using his own prolific fart production to scare off the Devil on numerous occasions.

Geoffrey Chaucer (c. 1343-1400) was a master storyteller, one of his most famous and humorous tales involving farting is that of *The Millers Wife*.

The Fart Side: Blowing in the Wind!

Rodin's "The Stinker"

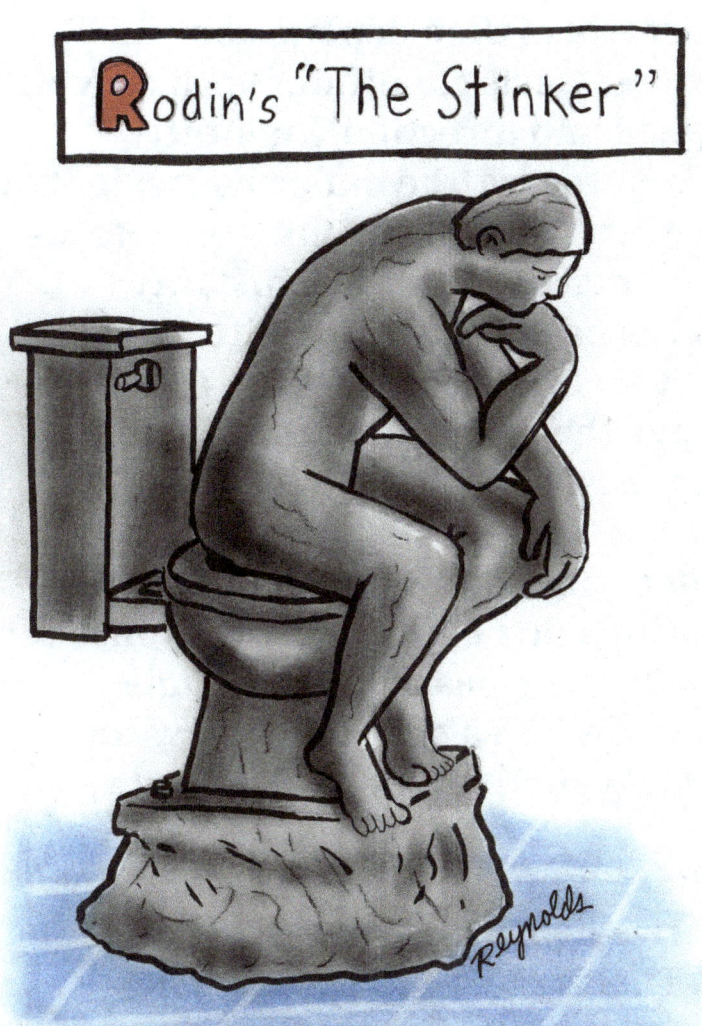

The Funny Side Collection

Fart travel time depends on atmospheric conditions such as wind speed and direction, humidity, temperature, the molecular weight of the fart particles including odorants and microbes, and the distance between the fart transmitter and the fart receiver. Farts diffuse as they leave the source, and their potency diminishes with distance.

There are conditions that exist for optimal fart odor concentration when the fart is released into a small enclosed area such as an elevator, small room, car, or shower stall.

There is often a several second delay between hearing a fart and smelling it. This is due to sound traveling much more rapidly than the aroma.

The Fart Side: Blowing in the Wind!

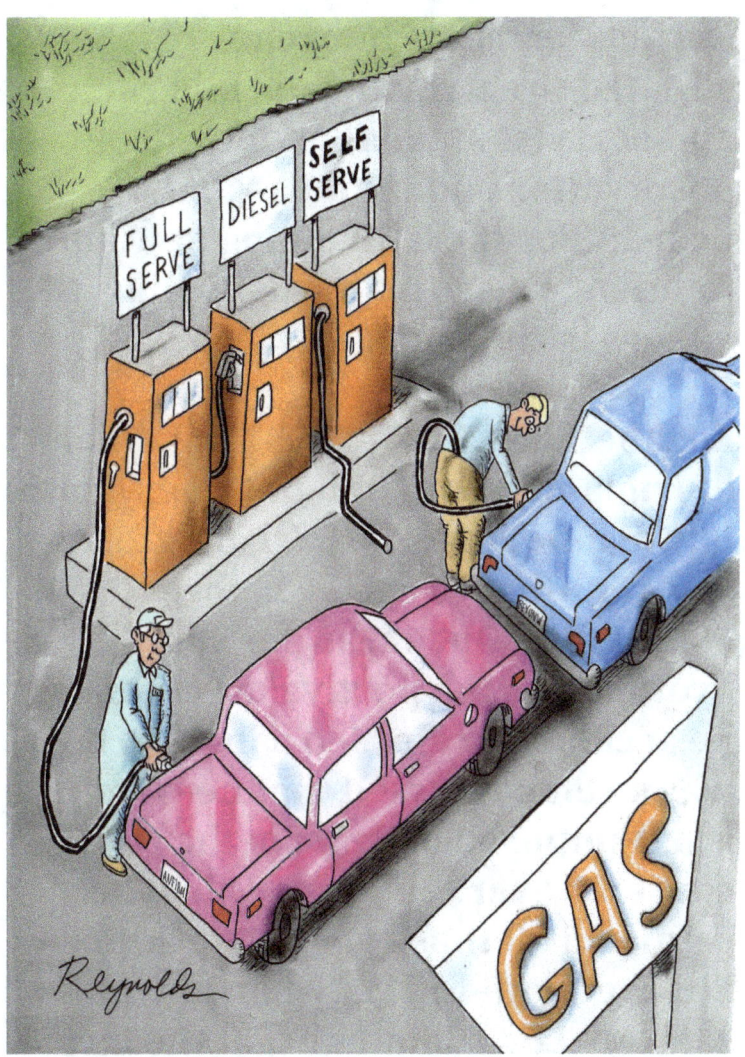

The Funny Side Collection

Lucius Mestrius Plutarchus (c. 46 – 120 AD) Greek historian, biographer, and essayist made the following observations about pulse and beans: "For the fruit, being new and flatulent, raises many disturbing vapors in the body."

Elizabeth I (1533 – 1603) was Queen of England from 1558 until her death. Edward DeVere, the Earl of Oxford, was required to curtsy before Her Majesty the Queen, as per court protocol. As the portly Earl curtsied, he accidently released a loud fart. He was so embarrassed that he went into a self-imposed exile from the royal court for over ten years. When he returned all those years later Queen Elizabeth offered a sly pardon and said 'My Lord, I hath forgot the fart".

The Fart Side: Blowing in the Wind!

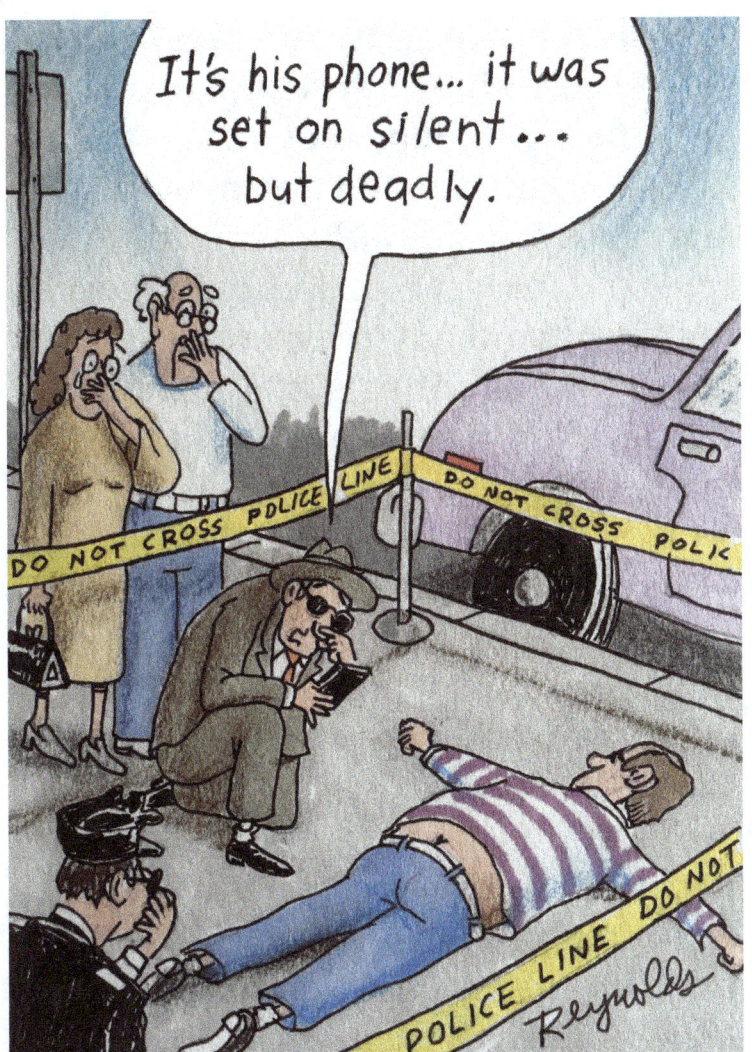

The Funny Side Collection

It is possible to capture a fart in a sealed container. The capture of a fart bubble underwater, into a water filled jar held upside down, holds a fart not exposed to the air until released later. To properly preserve the fart, avoid any reaction of sulfur based gasses with glass, plastic, or rubber. The container should be made of pure polypropylene.

The female southern pine beetle releases a pheromone, a hormone that serves as an olfactory sexual attractant, called frontalin in her flatus. It serves to attract males, but also attracts other females to engage with the males who respond. Predators are also attracted by the pheromone recognizing that it will lead to more prey.

The Fart Side: Blowing in the Wind!

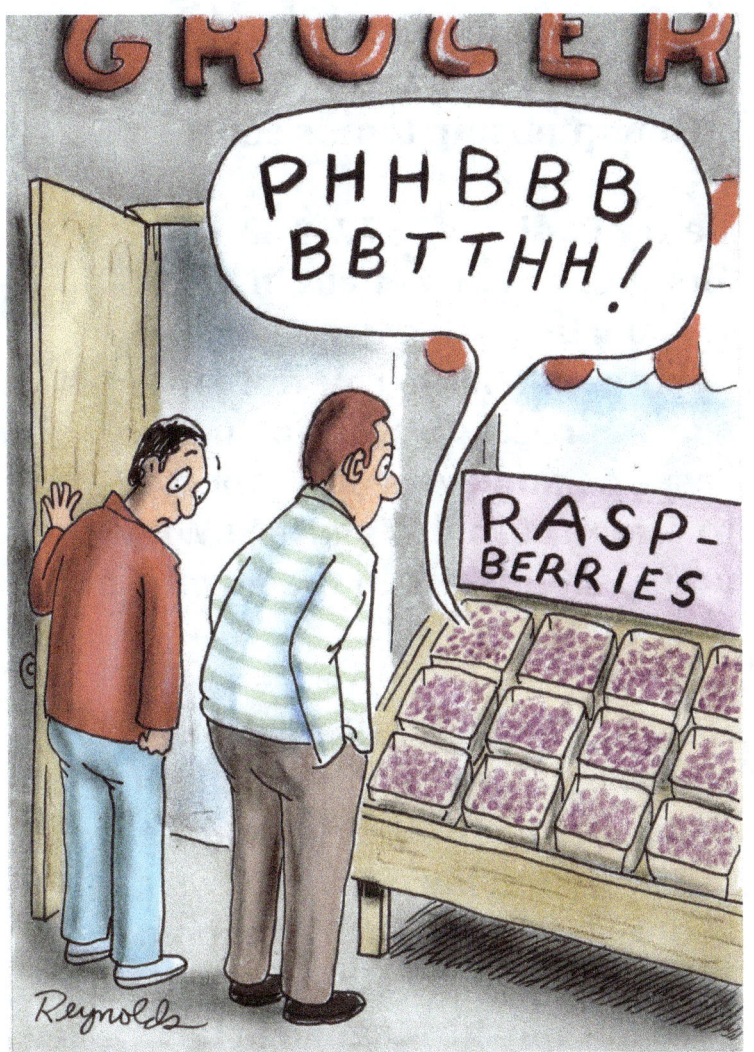

The Funny Side Collection

The surface area of the gastrointestinal tract exceeds that of a championship tennis court.

Henry Ludlow (1577–1639), a Member of Parliament in England was participating in a vigorous debate. When the roll call for votes was in process it was his turn to respond and everyone expected him to offer a resounding NAY! Which he unexpectedly did in the form of a loud fart.

Oliver Cromwell (1599-1658) was a controversial English leader who has been variously labeled as a regicide, dictator, and hero of liberty. Cromwell's derogatory response to a critic quoting the Magna Carta was "I care not for the Magna Farta".

The Fart Side: Blowing in the Wind!

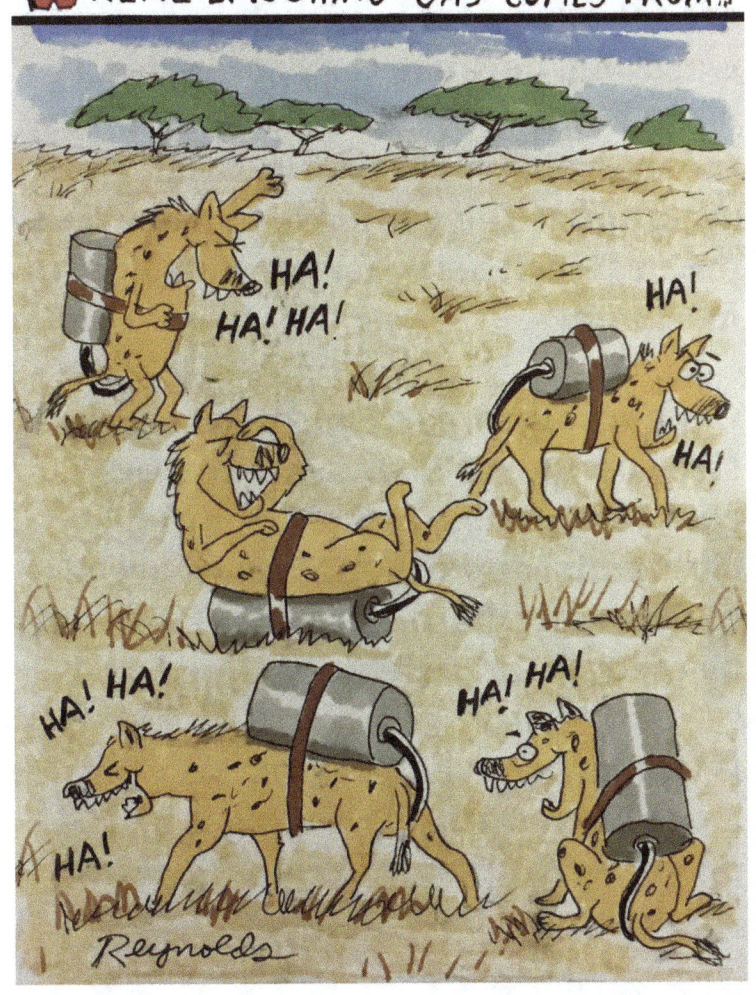

The Funny Side Collection

Termites are a major contributor to greenhouse gasses and global warming, because they comprise a large portion of the world's biomass, the microbes in their intestinal tract metabolize the cellulose in the wood they eat, releasing large quantities of methane.

Depending on herd and population size cows, pigs, sheep, horses, dogs, cats, kangaroos, camels, zebras, elephants, and other animals are also major contributors to global warming by farting and belching.

If you fart consistently for six years and nine months, enough gas is produced to create the energy of a small atomic bomb.

The Fart Side: Blowing in the Wind!

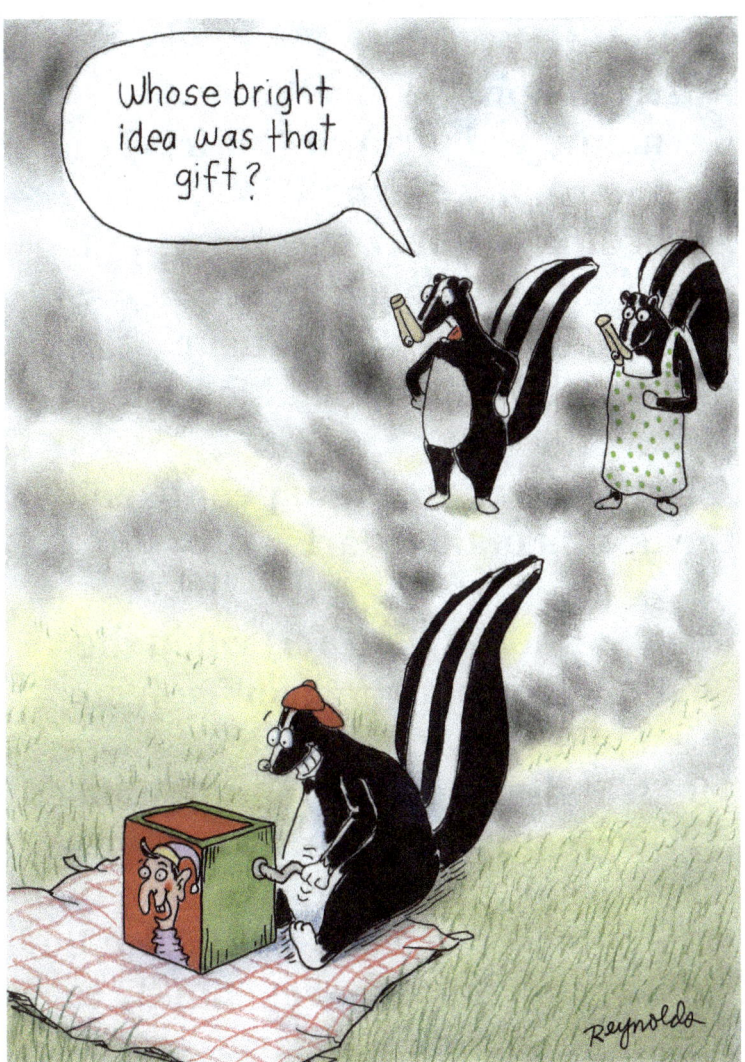

The Funny Side Collection

Adolf Hitler (1889 – 1945) was the Austrian born Chancellor of Germany, and dictator (Führer) of Nazi Germany during WWII. According to Pulitzer Prize winning historian and biographer John Toland, Hitler "suffered from meteorism, uncontrollable farting".

About thirty percent of people enjoy the aroma of their farts

Josef Stalin (1878-1953) ruled the Soviet Union with an iron fist from the mid-1920s until his death in 1953. Stalin had a profound phobia of farting in public. When attending meetings, he would always have two water glasses in front of him that he would clink together repeatedly to mask the sound of his farts.

The Fart Side: Blowing in the Wind!

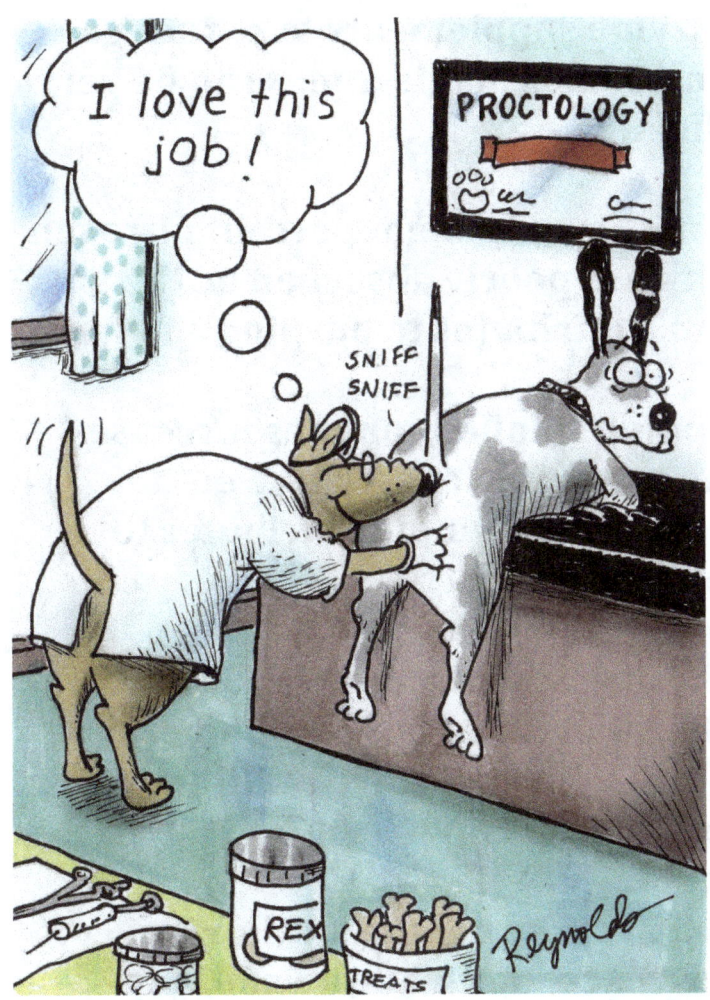

The Funny Side Collection

Enzyme supplements to reduce gas from beans and legumes can be very effective.

Air is seventy-eight percent nitrogen, which is poorly absorbed by the gut, and contributes to burping and farts.

Sipping smaller volumes increases the amount of air swallowed (aerophagia), and contributes to burping and farts.

The average person swallows two thousand times per day, and each swallow includes five milliliters (one teaspoon) of air.

The average person swallows every thirty seconds while awake, and every five minutes while asleep.

The Fart Side: Blowing in the Wind!

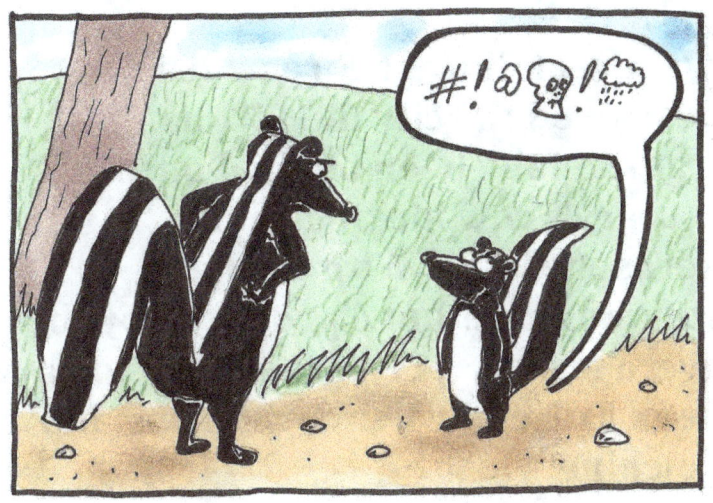

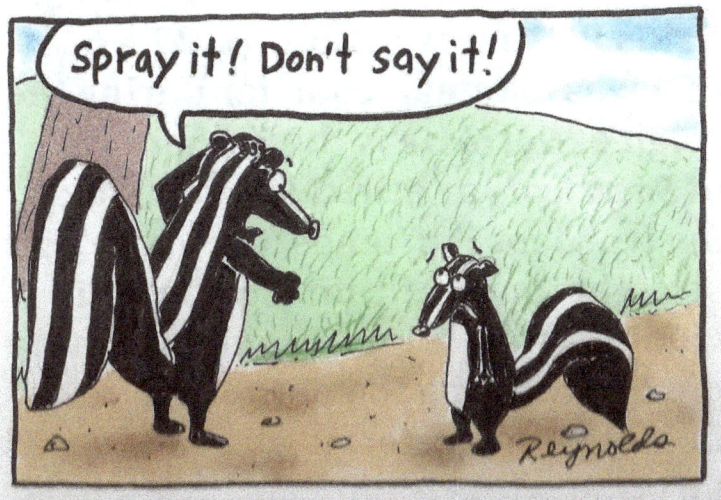

The Funny Side Collection

The Great Chicago Fire which destroyed the city in 1871 has traditionally been blamed on Mrs. O'Leary's cow kicking over a kerosene lamp. With the large volume of methane produced by the average cow, it is just as likely to have been caused by her cow farting and belching.

Gaius Petronius Arbiter (c. 27 – 66 AD) was a Roman courtier during the reign of Nero. He is the author of *Satyricon*, a satirical novel. "Take my word for it, friends, the vapors go straight to your brain. Poison your whole system. I know some who have died from being too polite and holding it in", referring to unreleased farts.

The Fart Side: Blowing in the Wind!

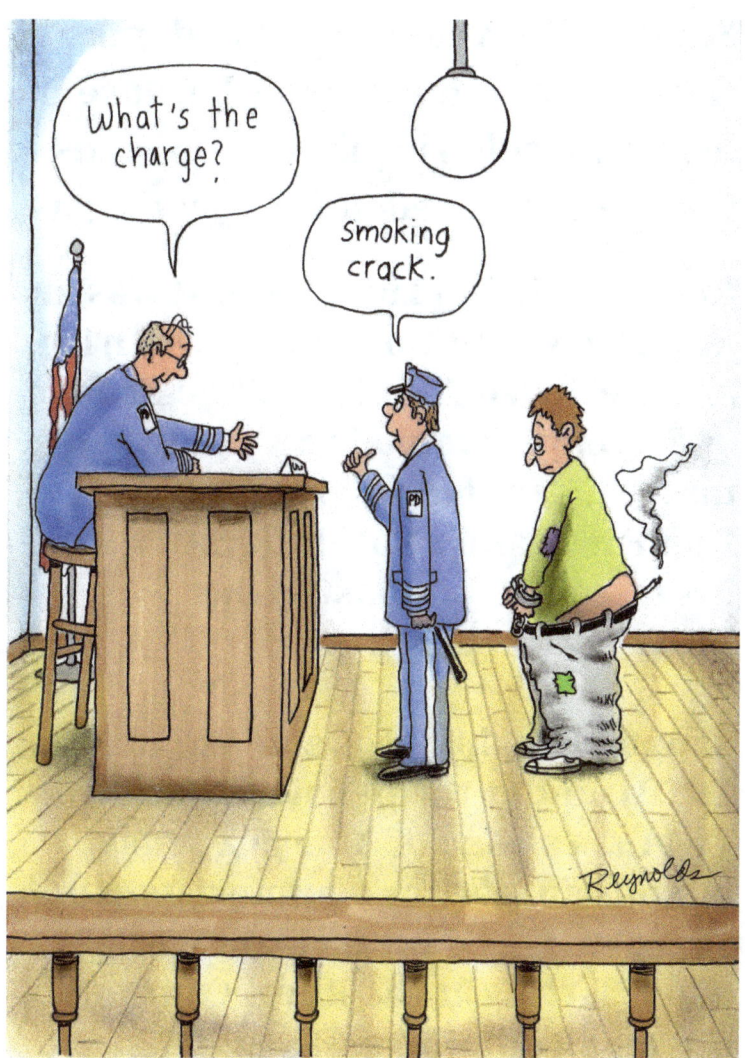

The Funny Side Collection

SCUBA divers cannot fart at depths of thirty-three feet or below because the high atmospheric pressure exceeds the pressure needed to expel the gas.

Jonathan Swift (1667 – 1745) was an Anglo-Irish author, essayist, satirist, and cleric. The pamphlet *The Benefit of Farting Explained* was published under his puffed-up pseudonym of Don Fartinando Puff-Indorst, Professor of Bumbast at the University of Crackow.

Samuel Langhorne Clemens (1835 - 1910), under the pen name Mark Twain, was one of America's most famous authors and humorists. His short story *1601* is a ribald work about farting at the Royal Court of Queen Elizabeth I of Great Britain

The Fart Side: Blowing in the Wind!

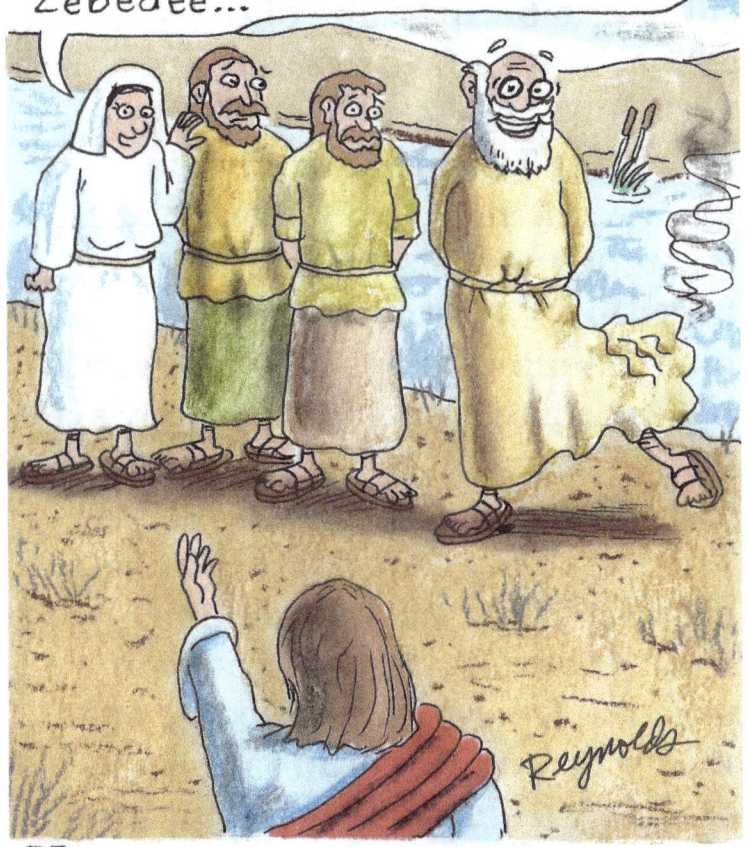

How James and John became known as "Sons of Thunder".

The Funny Side Collection

Roald Dahl (1916-1990) was an English novelist, poet, and fighter pilot who became one of the 20th century's favorite authors of children's books. In *The BFG* the character The Big Friendly Giant engages in an activity described as whizzpopping, the passing of intestinal gas, at formal events. The giants believe burps are disgusting, but farts are entertaining and they love farting.

The Russian words for fart include *perdyozh* (first act of breaking wind), *perdun* (perpetrator and outcome), *perdil'nik* (place from where it comes), *Perun* (ancient God of wind), *bzdun* (silent fart), and bzdyukha (silent fart, as well as a stupid jerk).

The Fart Side: Blowing in the Wind!

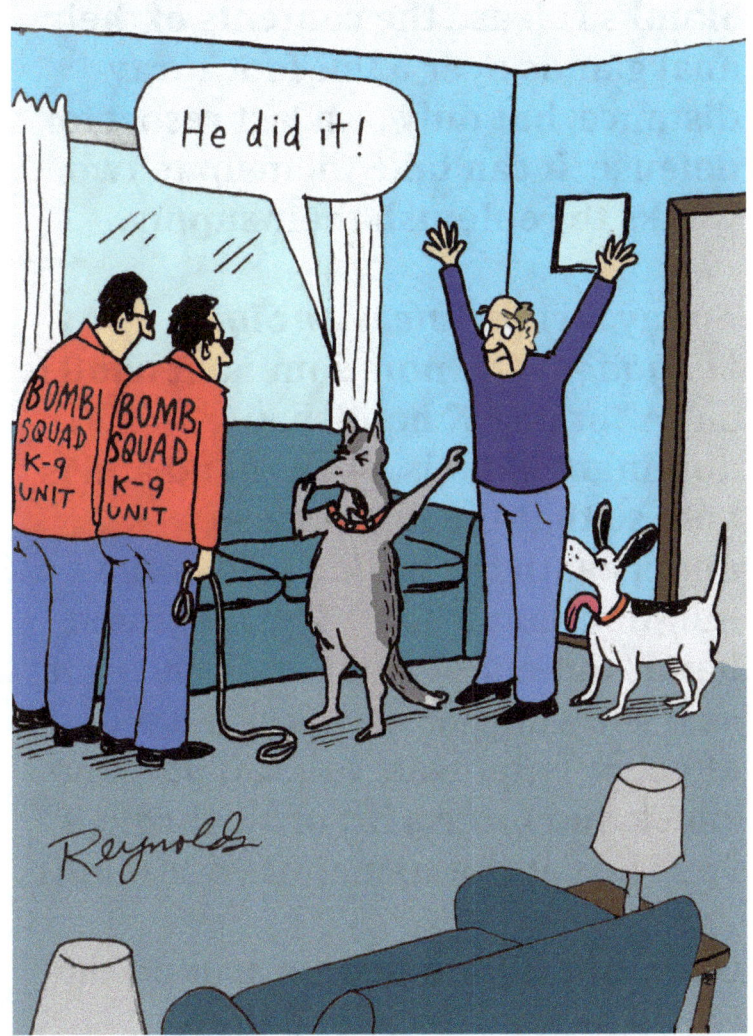

The Funny Side Collection

Skunks release the contents of their anal glands over a ten-foot spray distance, but only as a last resort for defense. It can take them up to two weeks to replenish their supply.

To say fart in *American Sign Language:* The non-dominant hand is an "A" or an "S" handshape. The dominant hand is a bent hand and is held so that the fingers are underneath the pinkie side of the non-dominant "fist." The dominant hand "unbends" and bends one time as if showing gas escaping. For comic effect or emphasis, you can puff one cheek and force a bit of air through your lips at the corner of your mouth.

Over four billion people around the world never use toilet paper.

The Fart Side: Blowing in the Wind!

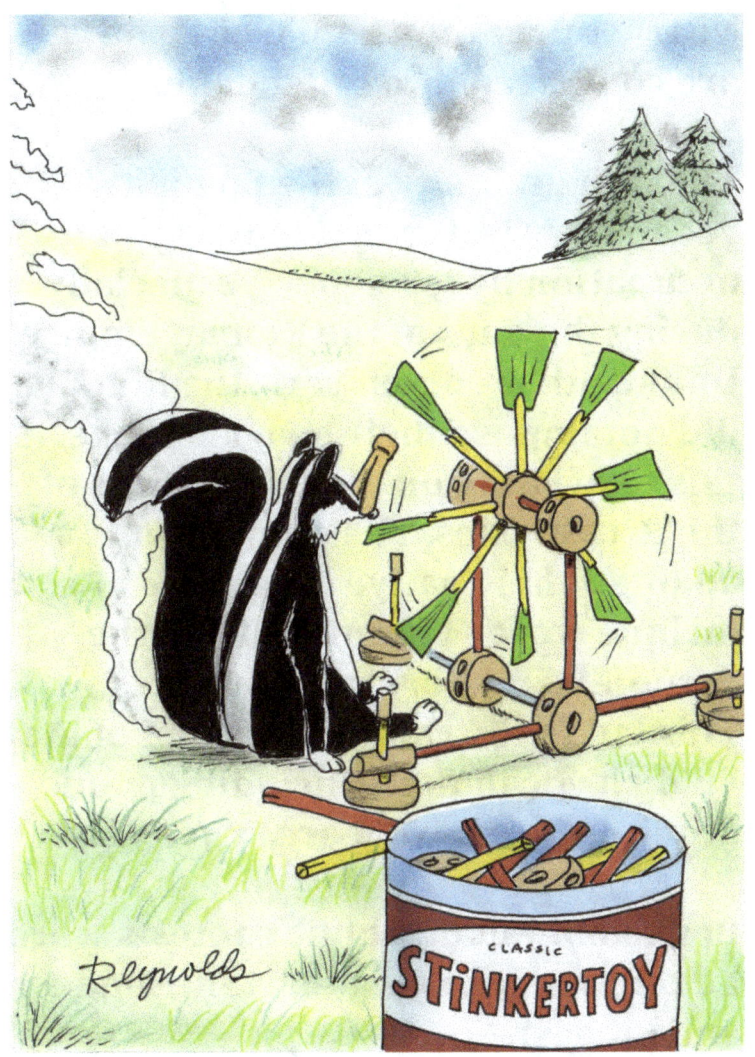

The Funny Side Collection

Nearly thirty thousand trees a day are converted into toilet paper.

The rich diversity of the English vocabulary is due to its history of occupation by foreigners, especially during the days of the Roman Empire. Unlike other conquerors, the Romans did not impose their own language, in this case Latin, on the inhabitants of the British Isles. The population adapted their native tongue to include words borrowed from the occupiers and foreign influences. This led to the rapid expansion of the English vocabulary, including many different words that are synonyms.

In ancient Japan, public contests were held to see who could fart the loudest and longest.

The Fart Side: Blowing in the Wind!

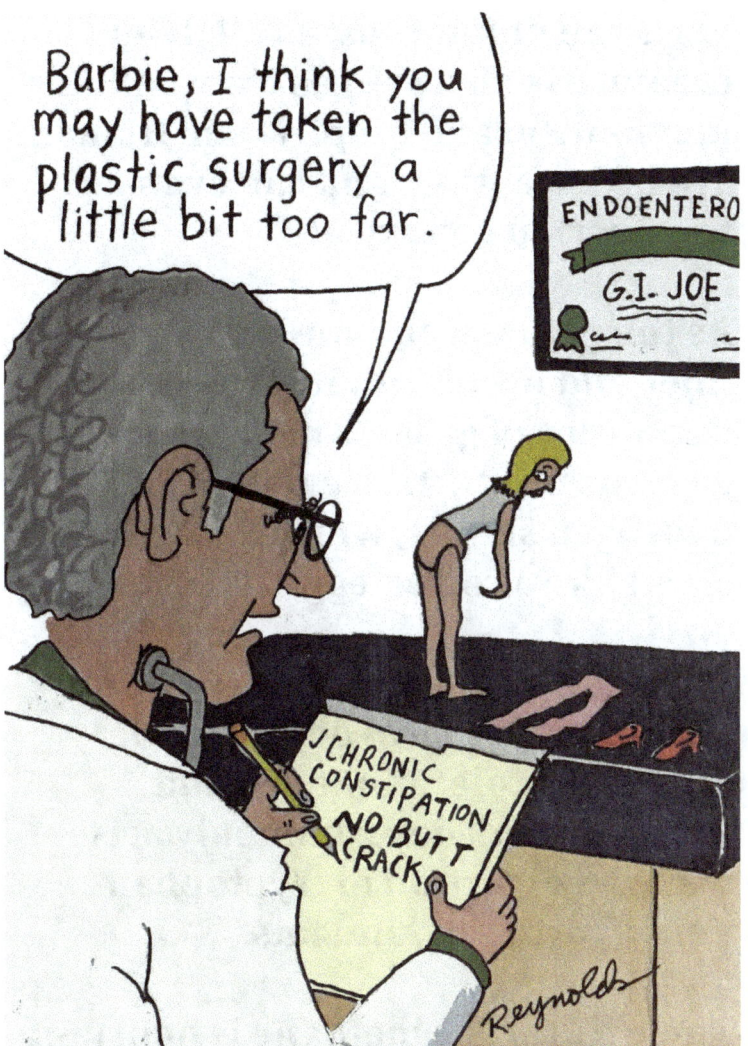

The Funny Side Collection

Farts are ubiquitous, as all living creatures generate gas from cellular metabolism and respiration. Humans are no exception, and can even fart for a period after death.

As the gut microbiome metabolizes fiber and prebiotics it generates vast quantities of gases. Among these gaseous products are odiferous hydrogen sulfide, which has a foul smell like a rotten egg.

Other gases that contribute to the characteristic fecal odor include indole, skatole, ammonia, and mercaptans. They commonly arise with the digestion of tryptophan, animal proteins, and fats.

The natural gas methane is odorless.

The Fart Side: Blowing in the Wind!

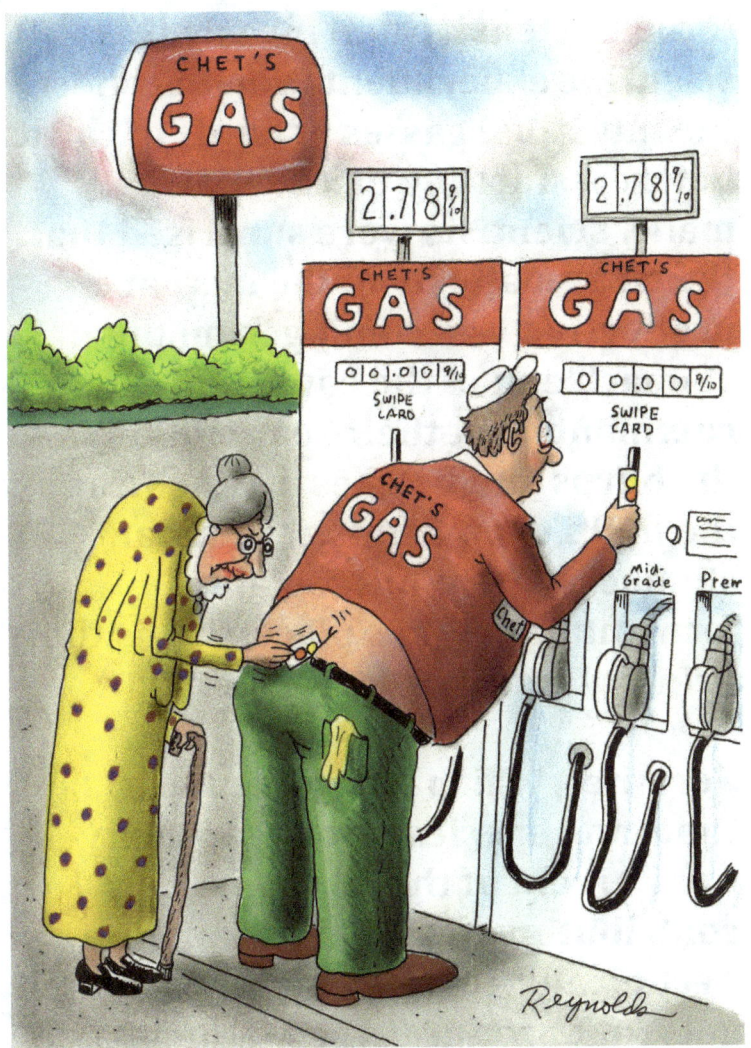

The Funny Side Collection

It took extensive and invasive scientific experimentation to collect the intestinal gasses of herds of cattle before a startling discovery was made. Scientists were surprised that the clear majority of the methane production was coming from the stomach end of the cows and other ruminants, not their rear ends. It is the burps and belches arising from the multi compartment ruminant stomach, where microbial fermentation takes place, that is the primary source of methane.

Termites, which have over two thousand species, produce twenty-five percent of the methane contributing to global warming. Technically, it is the microbes in their guts that produces the methane.

The Fart Side: Blowing in the Wind!

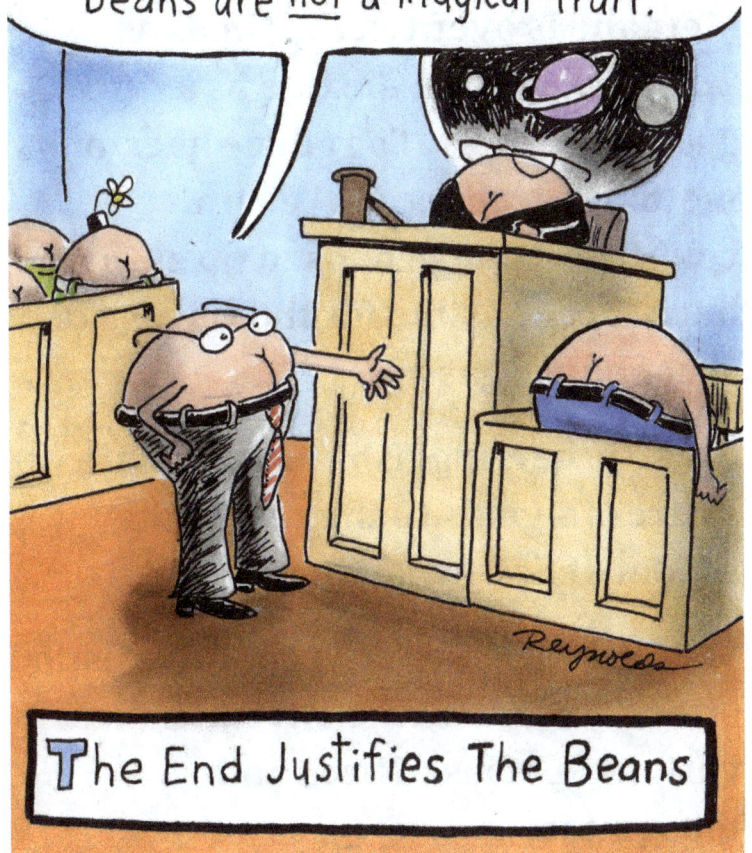

Ruminant bacterial fermentation is a significant contributor to global methane production.

Methane is over twenty times as potent as carbon dioxide as a greenhouse gas. To reduce livestock methane production, several countries have proposed taxes on the herds responsible for the release of greenhouse gasses.

Atlantic herring fish communicate distress signals to the rest of the school of fish by farting.

Skatole, which has the characteristic odor of feces, is attractive to males of various species of bees and mosquitos.

The Fart Side: Blowing in the Wind!

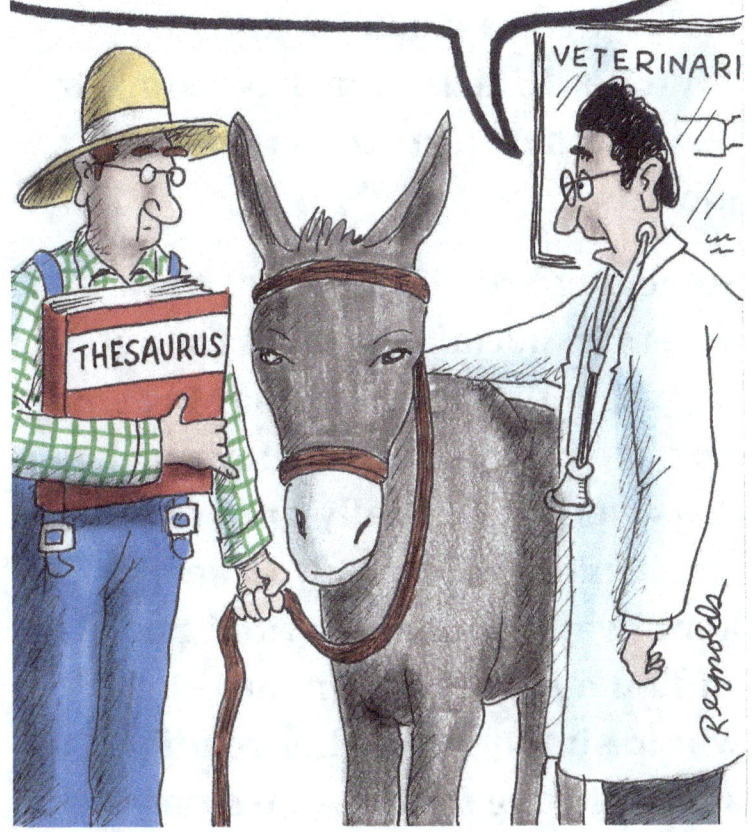

Dinosaurs have been accused of contributing to global warming. It is not known if they were ruminants, but there is no doubt that they were major farters. Their nickname "thunder lizards" may have more to do with their farts than their footsteps.

Some dog breeds fart more than others, especially the short snouted English bulldog and similar breeds that are regular air swallowers. Lap dogs were specifically bred to be small enough for a lady to keep with her always, and if intestinal gas ruffled her undergarments, she would simply blame her readily available dog for the emission.

The Fart Side: Blowing in the Wind!

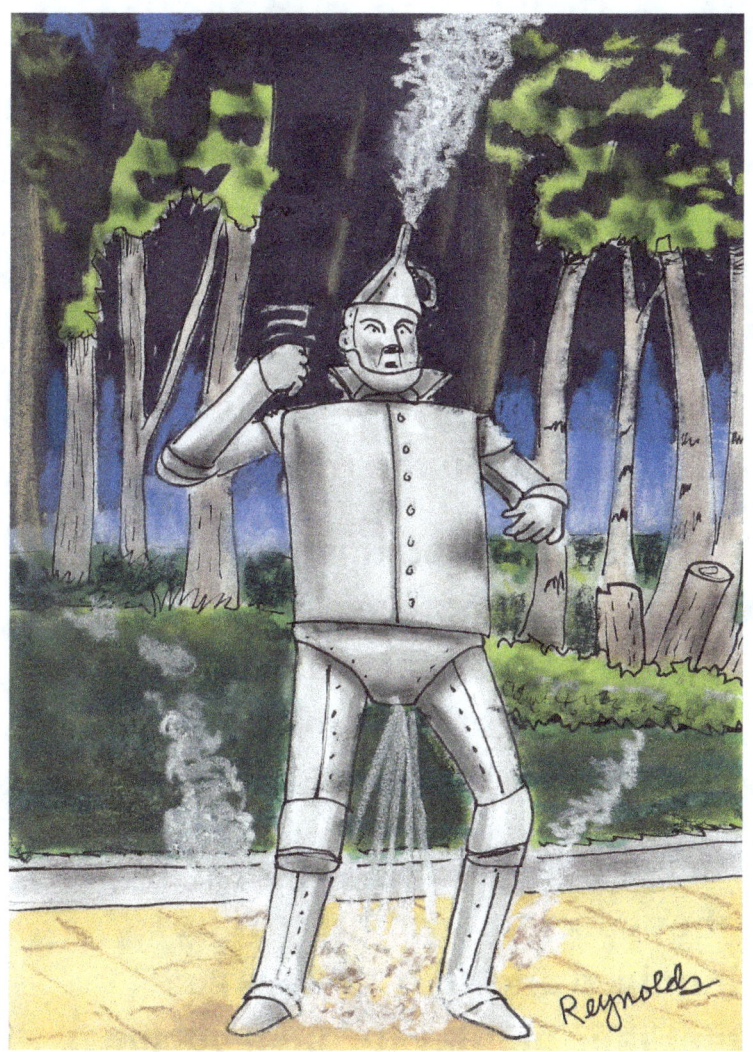

The Funny Side Collection

One third of Americans flush while still sitting on the toilet. This is very dangerous on aircraft and cruise ships where a powerful vacuum flush can lead to severe internal injuries if a tight seal occurs with sitting. There are forty thousand injuries a year while sitting on the toilet seat.

Termites trapped in amber, the petrified sap of trees, have preserved pockets of gas that still contain the methane that the termites passed hundreds to thousands of years ago.

An average cow is thought to release about six hundred liters (one hundred and sixty gallons) of methane per day through burping.

The Fart Side: Blowing in the Wind!

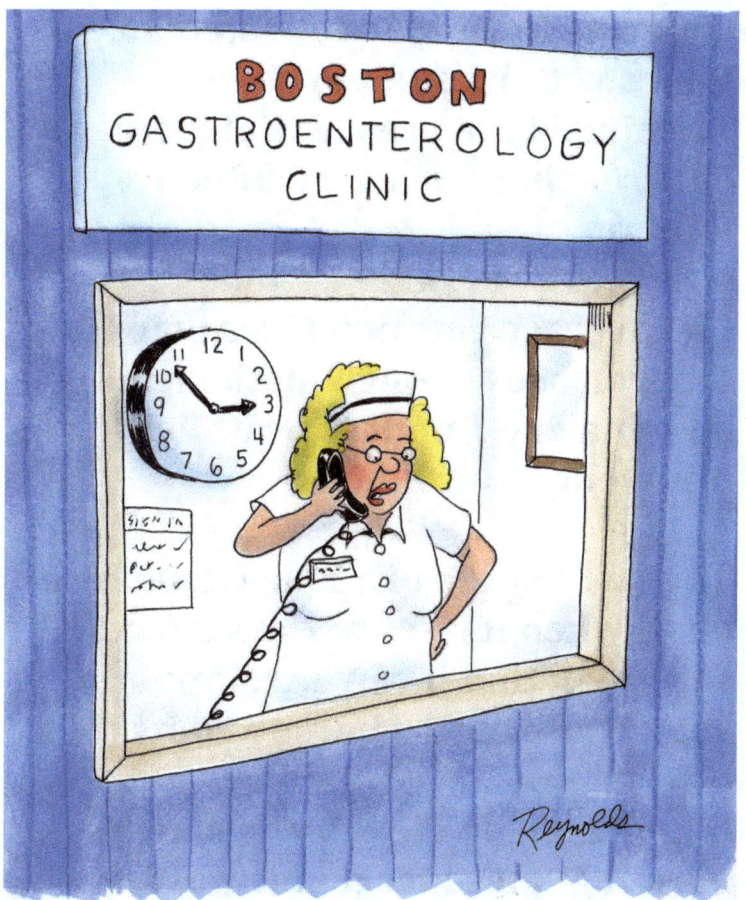

"No, I don't have an accent. I said your appointment was *too farty*."

The Funny Side Collection

Canaries were used for safety in coal mines with its sudden death a warning of the presence of methane. Cockroaches fart every fifteen minutes.

The average cow produces manure that releases enough methane to power a one-hundred-watt light bulb for twenty-four hours.

The fart bubble of a blue whale is so large when it rises to the surface of the ocean that it can envelope and asphyxiate both a horse and its rider.

Going up in an elevator in a high-rise building can cause an increase in farting because intestinal gasses expand as the atmospheric pressure decreases with ascent.

The Fart Side: Blowing in the Wind!

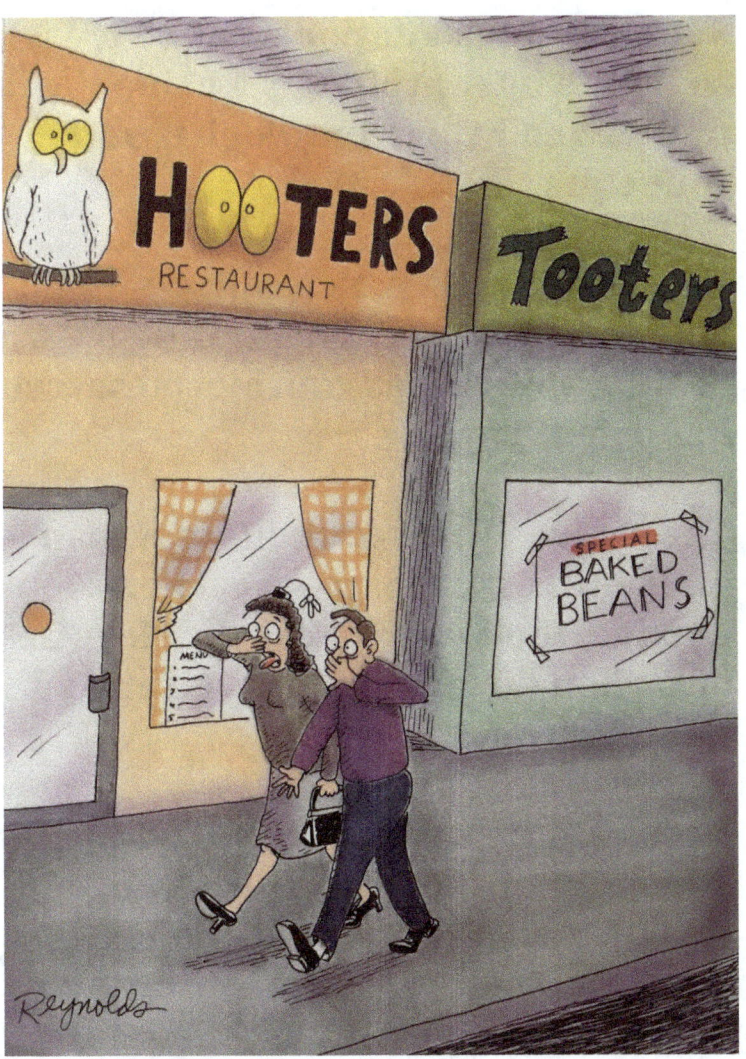

The Funny Side Collection

Petrified dinosaur poop, called a coprolite or coprolith, is a valuable find prized by paleontologists and collectors.

The dung beetle which collects animal droppings as a food and nesting source was considered sacred in Ancient Egypt.

The air we inhale contains less than one tenth of one percent carbon dioxide, the air we exhale has levels of carbon dioxide that is typically one hundred times as great.

These animals cannot fart: The Pogonophoran Worm, the Jellyfish and the Coral and Sea Anemones. This is a result of their anatomy, they do not have an anus.

The Fart Side: Blowing in the Wind!

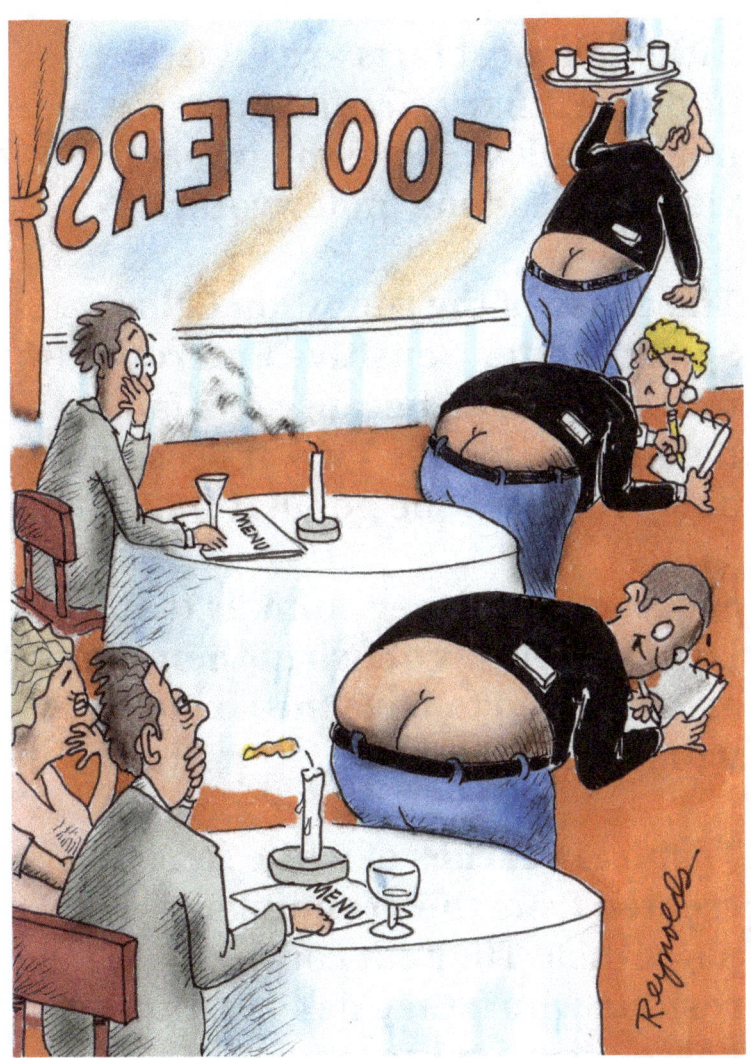

The Funny Side Collection

Although most farts are invisible under ordinary circumstances, it is not difficult to make them readily visible by farting underwater.

The cause of the condition Celiac Sprue (Gluten Sensitive Enteropathy) was discovered because of a famine during World War Two. It occurs in one percent of the population.

Sea lions and other animals that eat large quantities of fish in their diet are reported to have the world's worst smelling farts.

Tropical beaches of white sand are created from the droppings of the parrotfish. They eat coral, and the residue which they deposit after it passes as poop is considered sand.

The Fart Side: Blowing in the Wind!

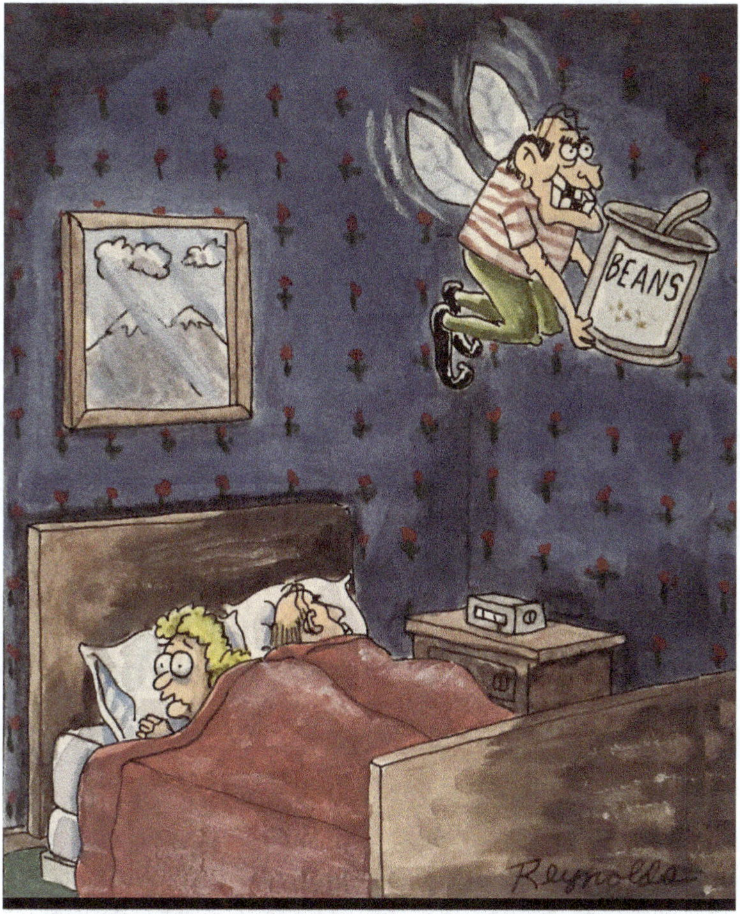
BEANS
Reynolds

Late at night, much to Mrs. Murray's dismay, Mr. Murray would often receive a visit from the "Toot Fairy".

The Funny Side Collection

Manatees control their buoyancy by farting when they want to submerge, and letting intestinal gasses build up when they want to float.

The Fitzroy River Turtle of Australia has the unique ability to also be able to breathe through its cloaca / anus.

A carminative is a preparation or herb that promotes the elimination of gas from the gastrointestinal tract. Many carminatives have been shown to work by releasing air swallowed (aerophagia) as a burp. A chocolate mint is a common carminative.

There are on average one hundred times more bacterial contaminants on restaurant menus than on restaurant toilet seats.

The Fart Side: Blowing in the Wind!

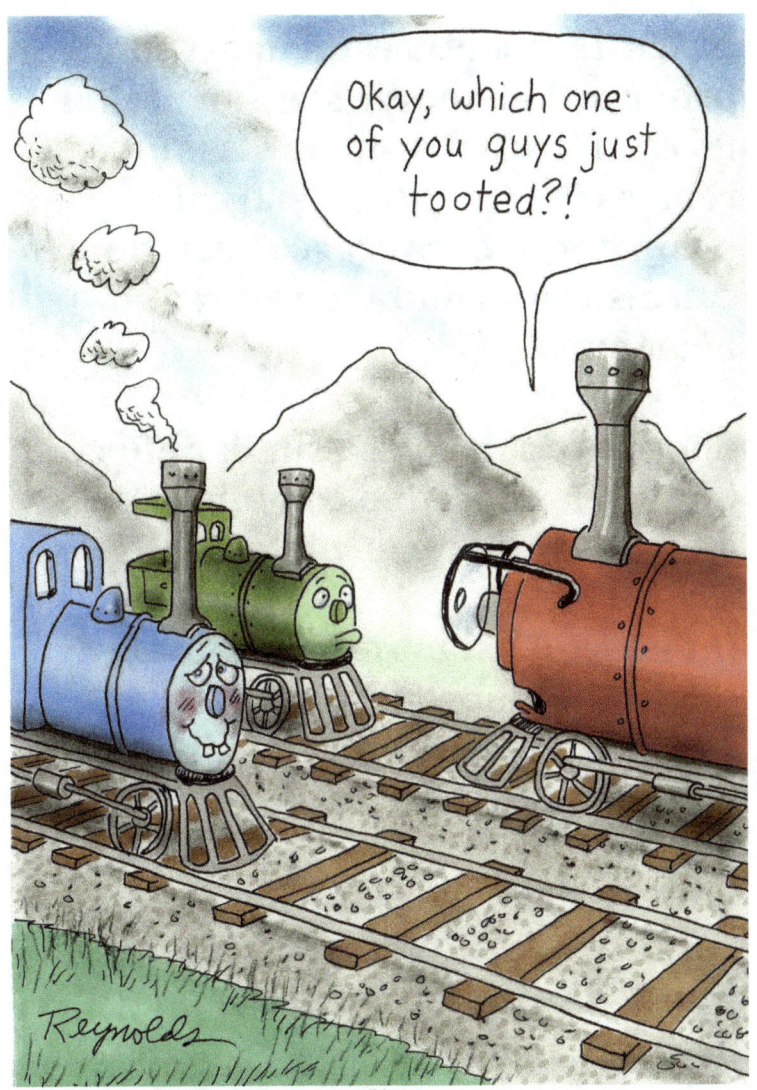

The Funny Side Collection

In Western culture, the most common product that people see and use for its carminative property is mint. It relaxes the lower esophageal sphincter to encourage eructation. It can also contribute to reflux and heartburn.

Chocolate can have a similar effect, so it is often offered in combination as an after-dinner chocolate mint.

Indian and Asian restaurants may offer other more traditional carminative herbs and seeds, usually found on the counter by the exit.

Women burp more during pregnancy because of the effect of hormones, as well as the increased abdominal pressure from the growing fetus.

The Fart Side: Blowing in the Wind!

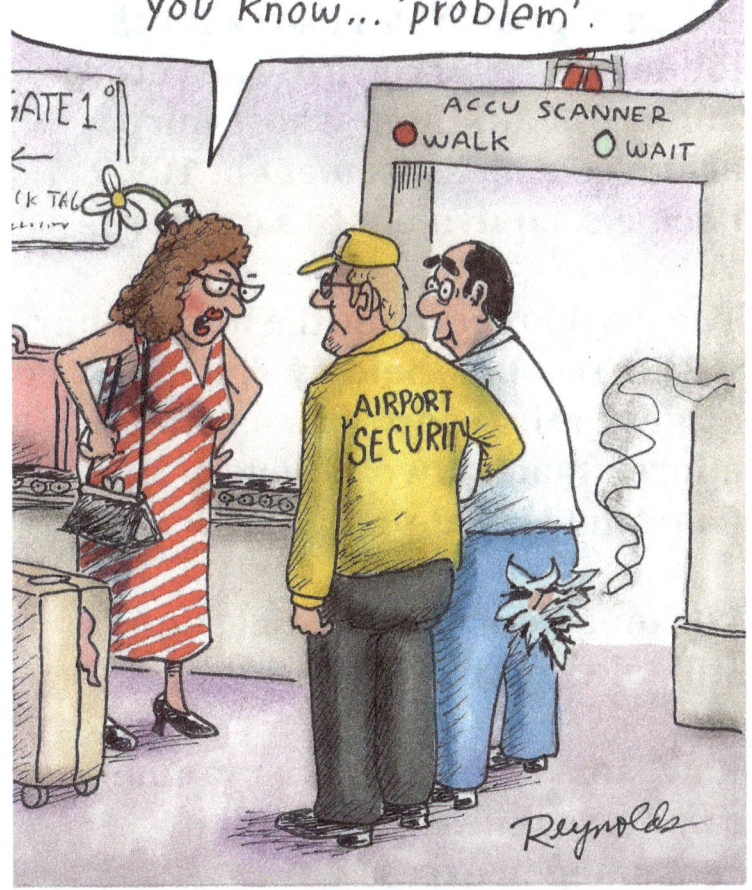

The Funny Side Collection

The World Burping Federation holds the annual World Burping Championship. The *Guinness Book of World Records* has a listing for the loudest burp on record. The record holder is Paul Hunn whose burp achieved a measurement of 109.9 decibels, equivalent to a car horn.

The world record for the longest burp is 18.1 seconds, held by Tim Janus. To achieve this record, he consumed approximately two gallons of Diet Coke and Mountain Dew.

Without stomach acid digestion can still take place.

Raw Lima beans contain cyanide and can cause illness and death if consumed in excess.

The Fart Side: Blowing in the Wind!

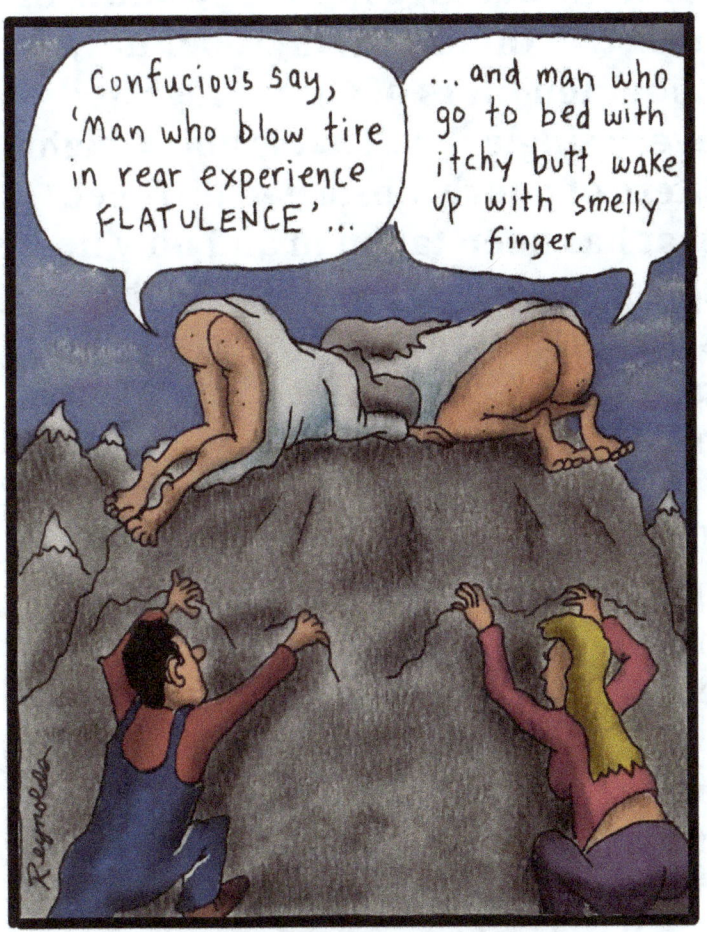

Wise Cracks

With the average human swallowing over two thousand times per day, about ten liters of air are ingested every single day. That is about eight liters of poorly absorbed nitrogen that has been taken in and now needs to get out. The most direct exit, the shortest distance to travel, and the fastest way to get relief, is to burp or belch.

That is much more gas than the most frequent and dedicated burpers and belchers are able to release through eructation. The retained nitrogen will contribute to bloating and distension, before it eventually makes its way out of the other end of the intestinal tract as a fart. Because of this, air swallowing (aerophagia) is a major contributor to farting.

The Fart Side: Blowing in the Wind!

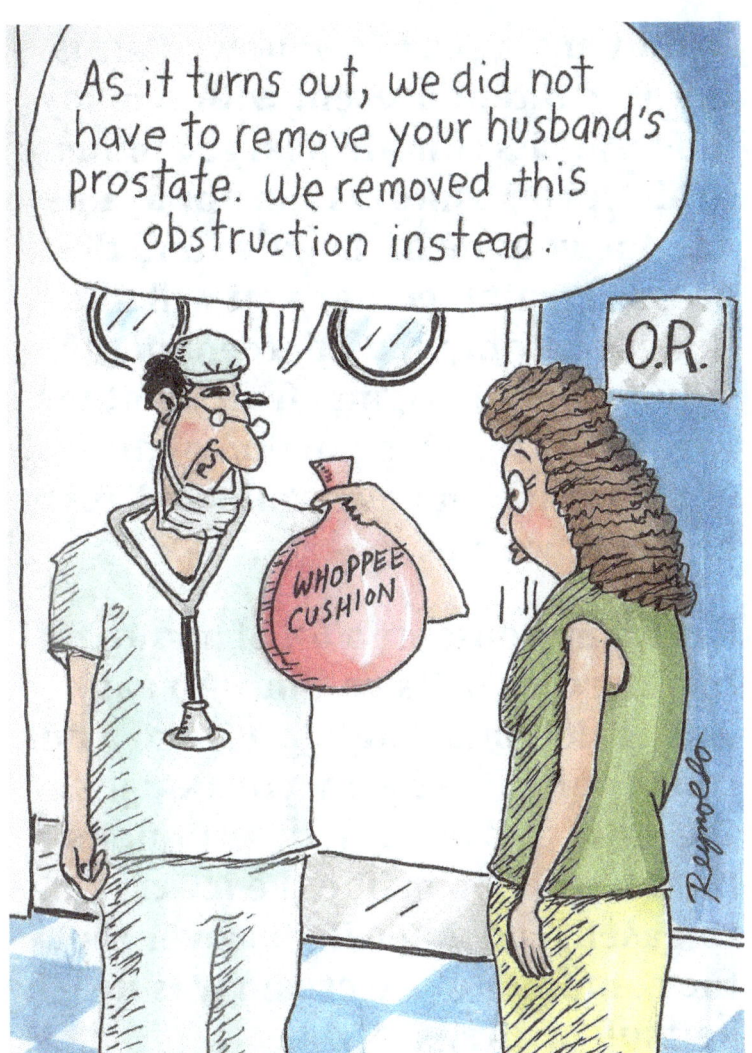

The Funny Side Collection

A hidden source of swallowed air is the air content present within many foods. Fruits contain a large amount of air. If you compress an apple and add the volume of the juice and the pressed fruit together you will find that it was only sixty percent of the volume of the original fruit. In other words, the missing portion of the entire fruit that you swallowed, forty percent, was air.

Ice cream contains a lot of air, up to fifty percent of its volume. An easy way to demonstrate this is take a full container of ice cream you bought at the store and let it melt. As it melts the air trapped inside the ice cream is released, and you will discover that the container of ice cream was nearly half full of air.

The Fart Side: Blowing in the Wind!

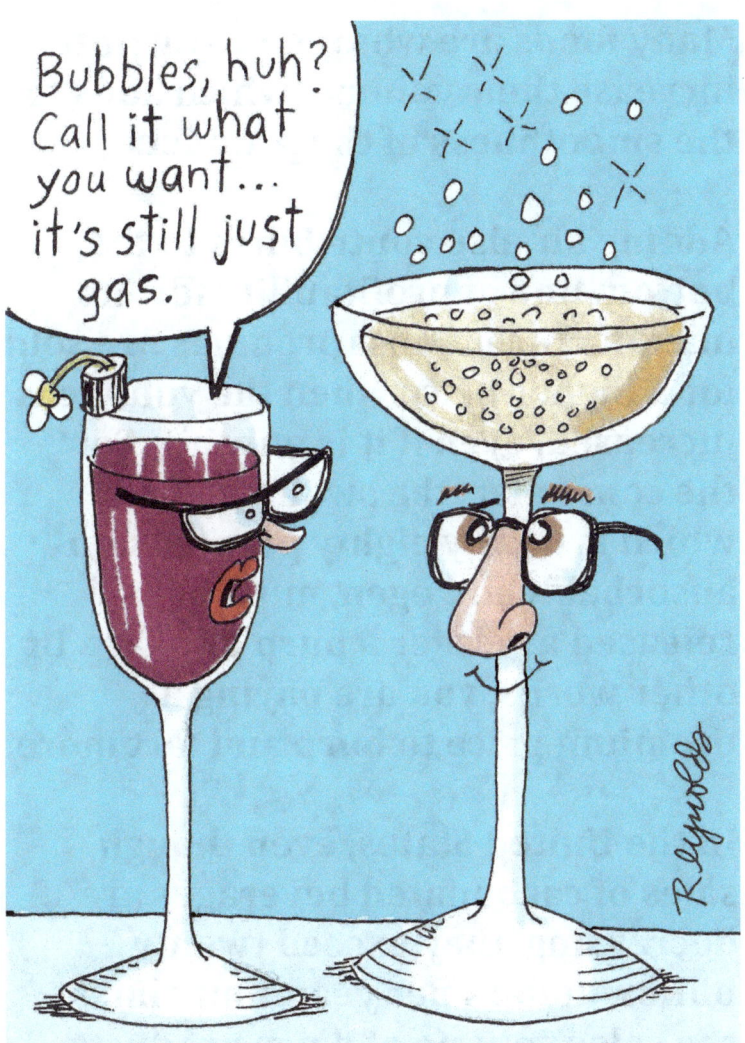

The Funny Side Collection

Many foods are whipped with air to increase their volume, which adds to the smoothness of the product.

Adding air also contributes to the bottom line of profitability for the manufacturer. Most products are sold for a higher price when the volume is increased, even if it is only air. For the consumer, the swallowed air, which is nearly eighty percent non-absorbable nitrogen, must be released as either a burp or a fart. In other words, you are paying a premium price to burp and fart more.

In the United States, even though sales of carbonated beverages are decreasing, they exceed twenty billion dollars per year, four times the sales volume of dairy products.

The Fart Side: Blowing in the Wind!

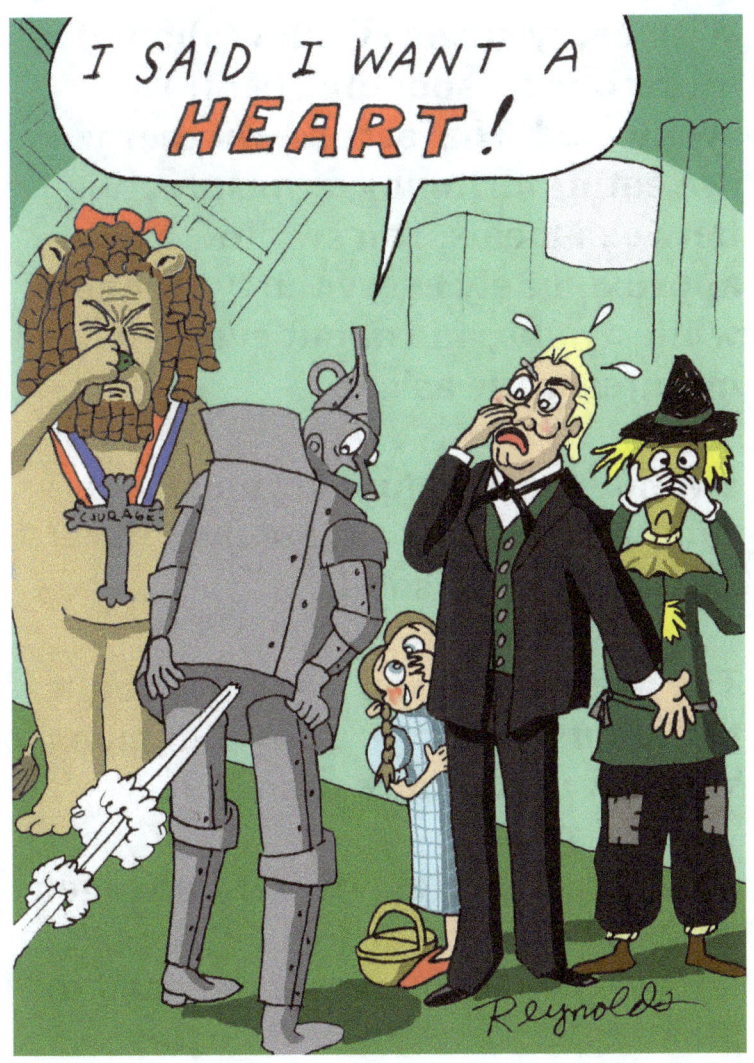

The Funny Side Collection

With every single swallow about five ml, or one teaspoonful, of air is swallowed. This occurs whether you are eating, drinking, or just resting between meals. You swallow approximately every thirty seconds while awake, and about every five minutes while asleep.

Swallowing of a liquid is more complex and challenging than the swallowing of a solid.

The average person swallows about two thousand times a day, but many swallow much more than that.

Air is seventy-eight percent nitrogen, which is a poorly absorbed gas. If it is not released in a burp, it will lead to bloating, distension, and farting.

The Fart Side: Blowing in the Wind!

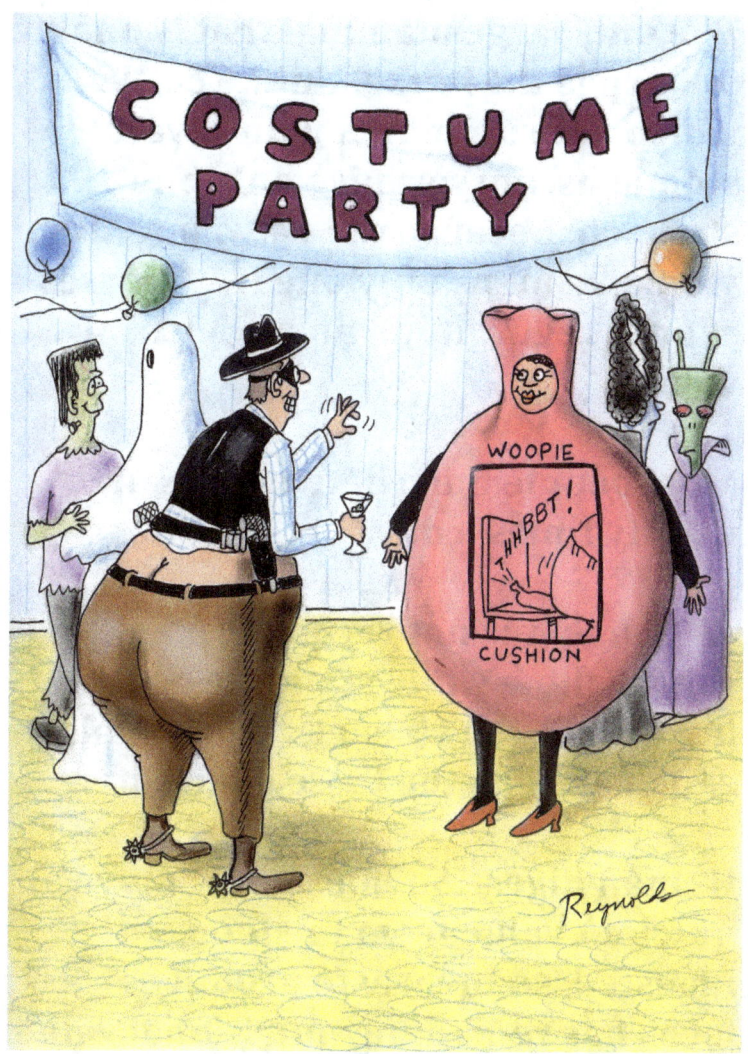

The Funny Side Collection

The only large mammal that is unable to burp is the horse. Unlike cattle which are ruminants with several stomachs, horses have only one stomach. Because the valve into the stomach opens only one way, horses cannot regurgitate, burp, belch, or vomit.

Most people burp between six and twenty times a day.

Although it is not recommended, you can swallow while standing on your head since the strength of peristalsis can overcome the force of gravity.

Human digestion does not remove all nutrient value from the food ingested, so the waste product of feces has remaining nutritional value.

The Fart Side: Blowing in the Wind!

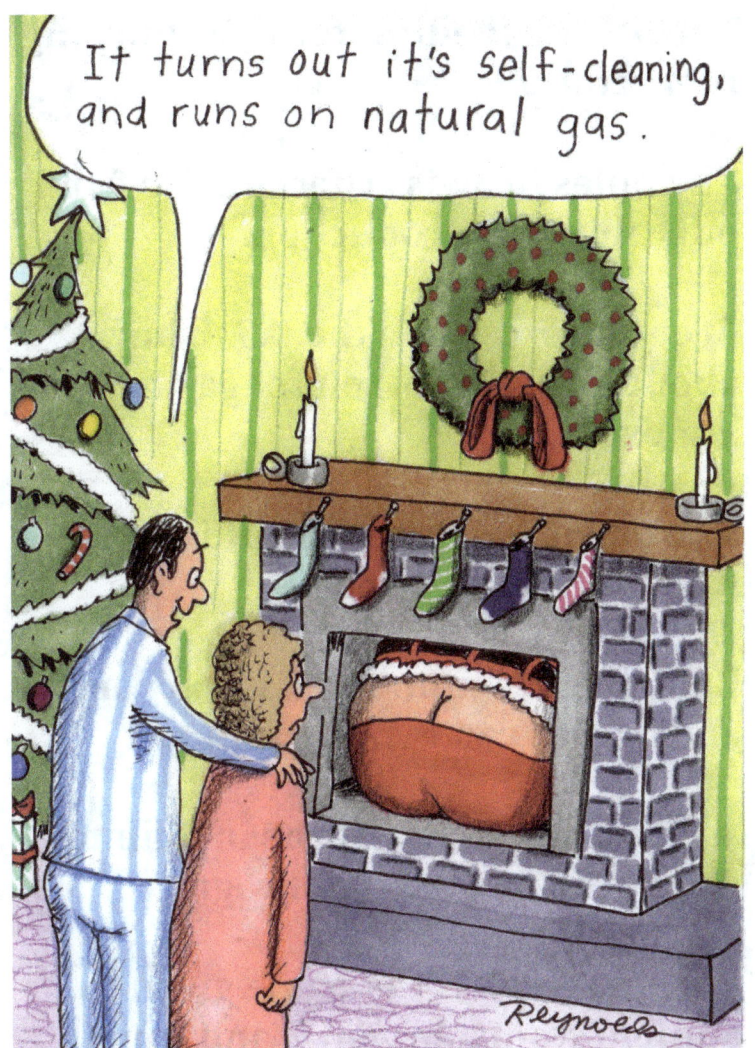

The Funny Side Collection

The official medical term for burping is eructation.

The holes in Swiss cheese arise from microbial gas production.

Every year cows in the U.S.A. burp about fifty million tons of gas into the atmosphere.

The burps of ten cows could heat a small house for a year.

Rats, rabbits, guinea pigs, chickens and horses can't vomit or burp.

A hiccup is caused by the involuntary contraction of the diaphragm.

Borborygmus is the name given to audible stomach growls and sounds.

The Fart Side: Blowing in the Wind!

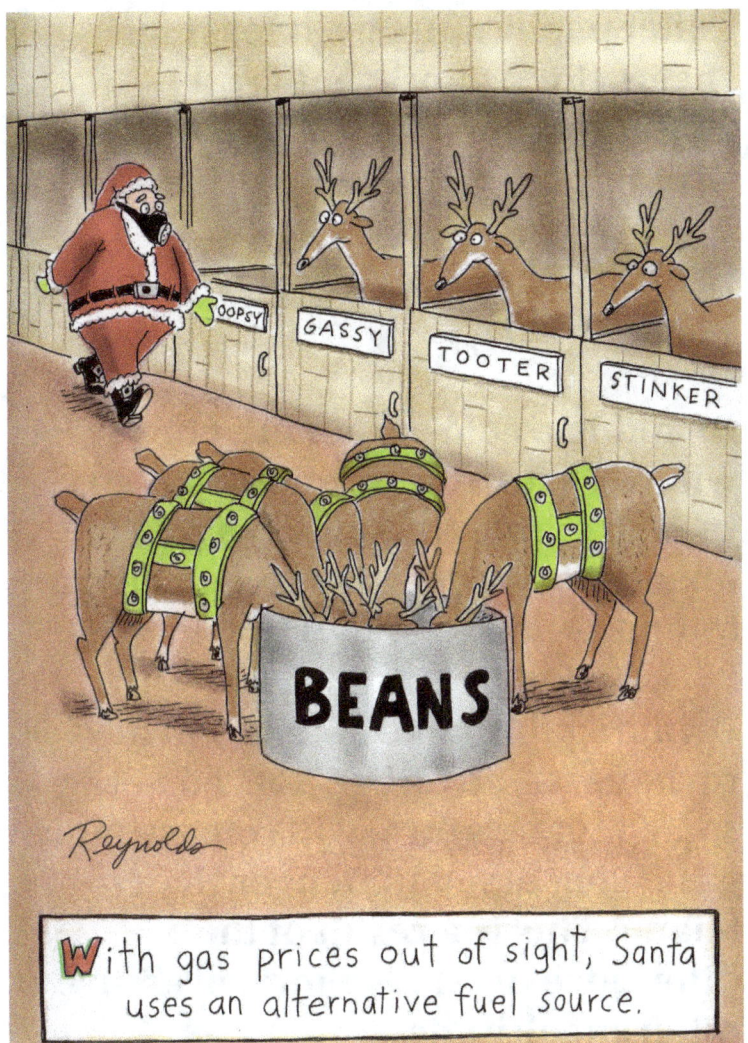

The Funny Side Collection

Toilet paper must be at least ten sheets thick to prevent fecal contamination of the hands with wiping.

Poor fitting dentures can contribute to intestinal gas.

Drinking a cold carbonated beverage will release greater volumes of gas than drinking the same type and quantity of beverage served at room temperature.

Drinking the same quantity of a carbonated beverage, served at the same temperature, will release more gas if consumed in Denver than in Miami. This is a result of the difference in atmospheric pressure at different altitudes.

The Fart Side: Blowing in the Wind!

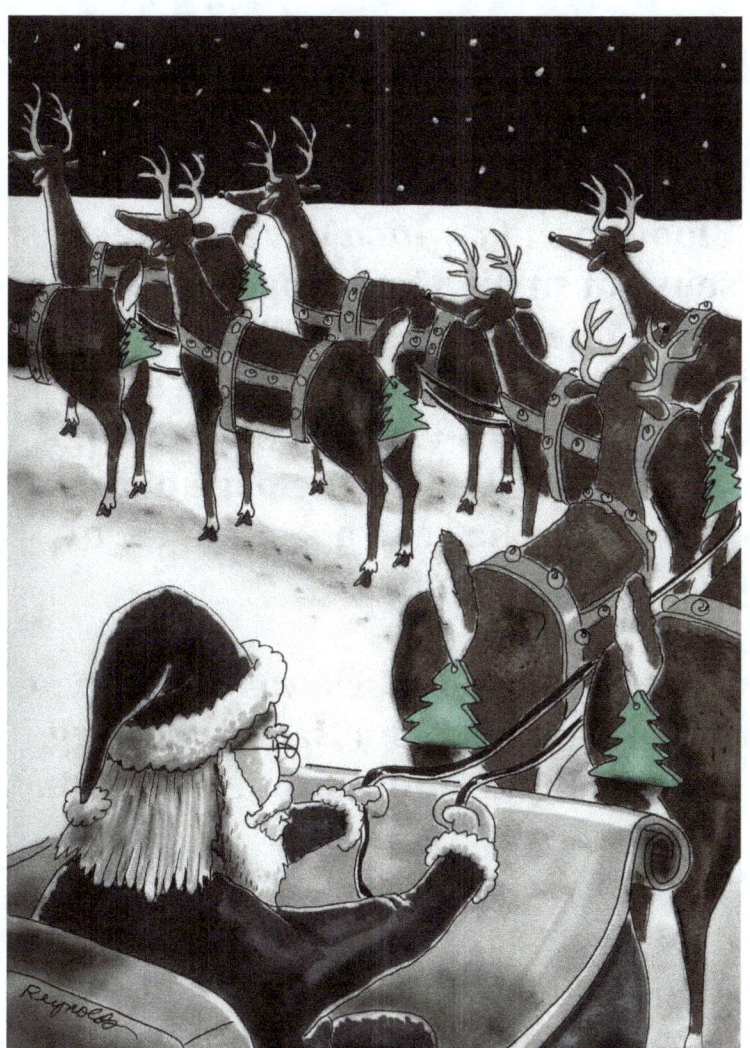

The Funny Side Collection

Carbonated beverages outsell dairy products by a ratio of four to one in the United States.

Bloodhounds, which have the keenest sense of smell of any dogs, have noses ten to one-hundred-million times more sensitive than a human's. Put into terms of a visual acuity analogy, it is as if the text on the page of this book could be read at a distance of two thousand miles.

Kellogg's Corn Flakes was developed by a physician, John Harvey Kellogg, specifically to address bowel health.

Graham Crackers were developed by a minister as a food with high fiber and roughage that was thought to aid in the suppression of masturbation.

The Fart Side: Blowing in the Wind!

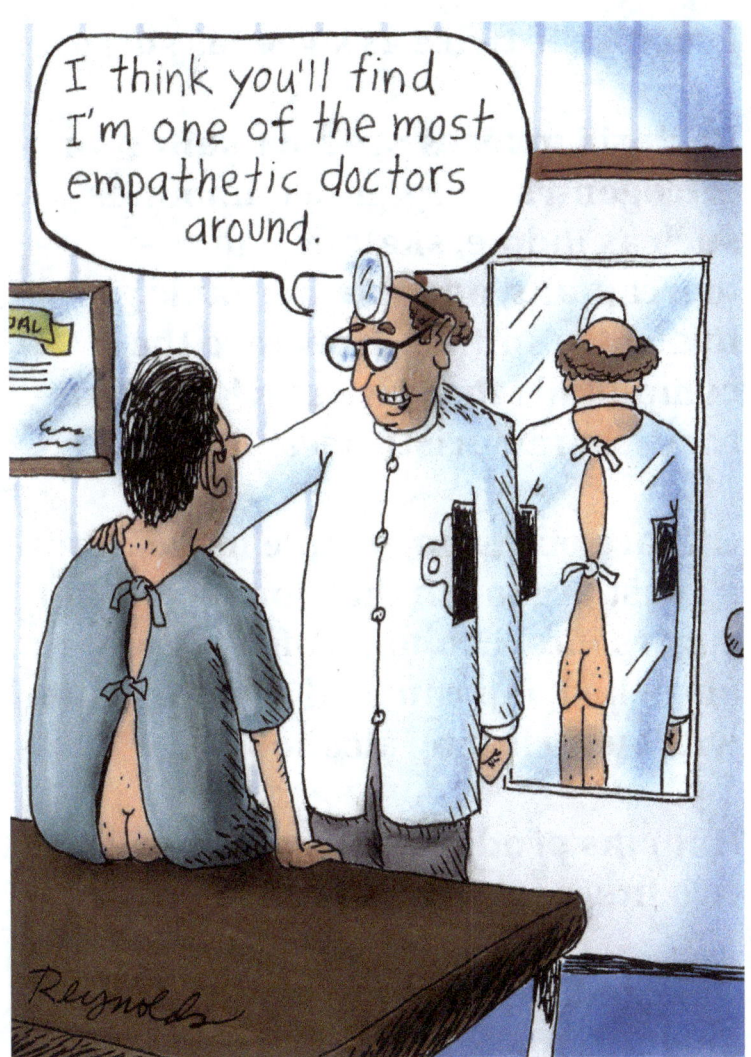

The Funny Side Collection

Fructose is twice as sweet as sucrose.

Bacteria in feces produce sulfur- or nitrogen-rich organic compounds such as indole, skatole, and mercaptans, and the inorganic gas hydrogen sulfide. These are the compounds that give stool and farts their characteristic fecal odor.

On rare occasion, people may harbor a yeast organism that converts plant sugars into alcohol, which is then absorbed and can lead to intoxication without drinking alcohol.

Humans produce on average one to two liters (quarts) of saliva per day.

The medical term for swallowing is deglutition.

The Fart Side: Blowing in the Wind!

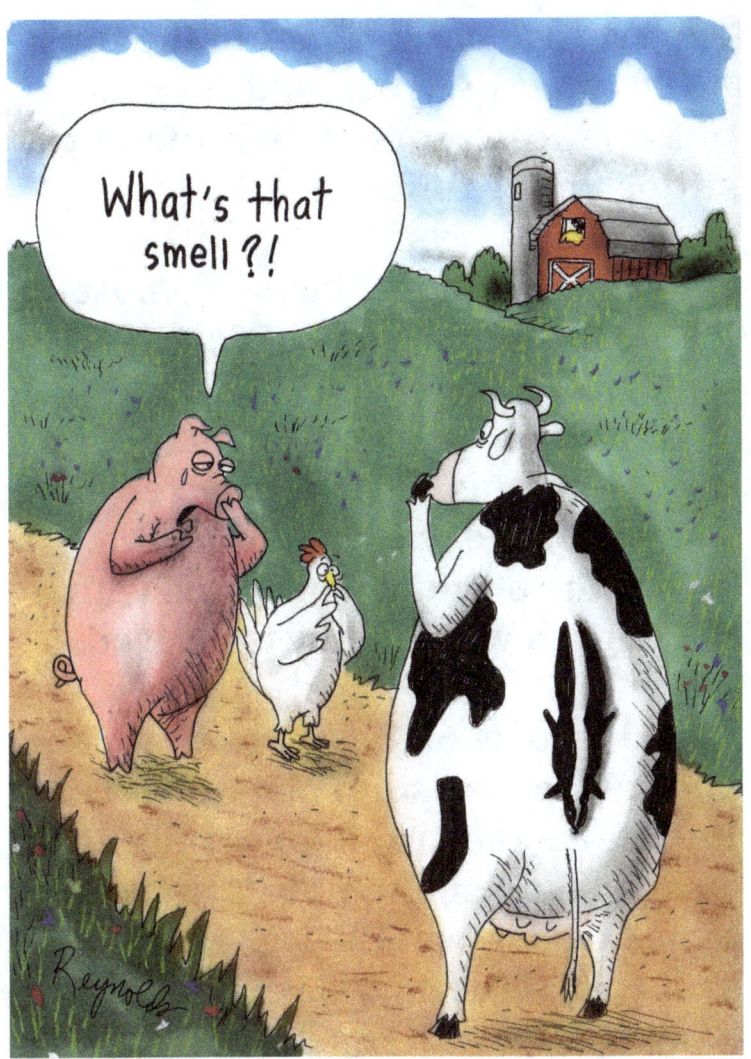

The Funny Side Collection

The average person goes to the toilet 2,500 times per year, and spends a total of three years of their lifetime sitting on the toilet.

For those musically inclined, most toilets flush in the key of E flat.

Sugar cane was processed in India over two thousand five hundred years ago, and was called khanda. This is the original word from which the English word candy is derived.

In many parts of the world, popular and religious custom dictate that only the left hand be used for wiping after a bowel movement. This is believed to be the origin of the right-hand shake as a greeting, since the left hand was considered unclean.

The Fart Side: Blowing in the Wind!

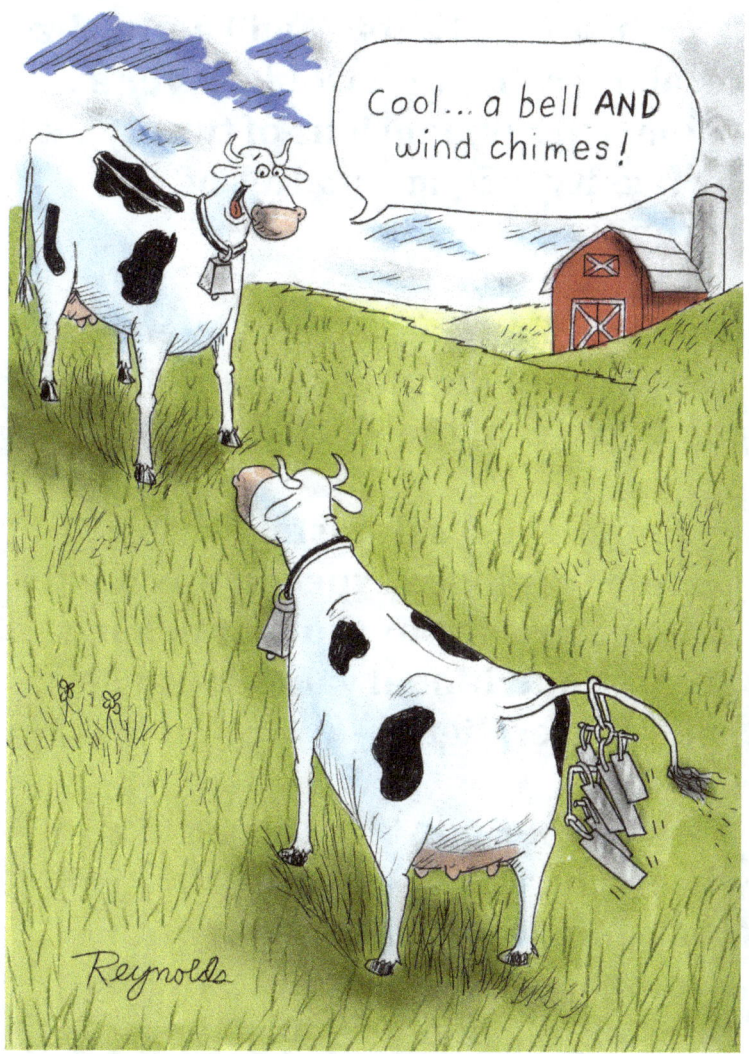

The Funny Side Collection

The flushing of a toilet will aerosolize fecal microbes that would cover a room, with dimensions of twenty feet by twenty feet, in a matter of seconds.

The use of human feces as a fertilizer, known as night soil, is common in many parts of the world.

In Japan, the fecal waste of rich people was more expensive as night soil because it was thought to have greater nutritional value, because of their better diet.

Toilet paper must be at least ten sheets thick to prevent fecal contamination of the hands with wiping. This is why toilet paper is inferior to a bidet for hygiene.

The Fart Side: Blowing in the Wind!

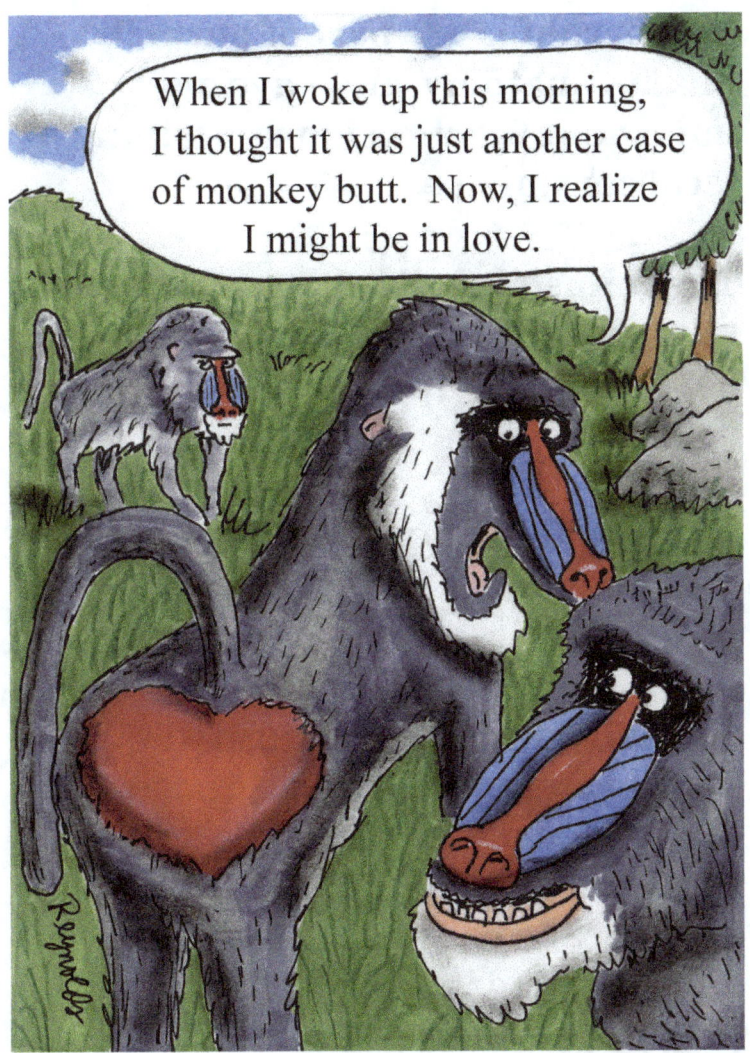

The Funny Side Collection

Hemorrhoids are part of normal human anatomy, and have an important function in maintaining fecal continence.

Toilet flush handles have over four hundred times as many fecal bacterial contaminants as the toilet seat.

More than twenty-five billion rolls of toilet paper are sold every year in the U.S.

Specially designed toilets in the space shuttle and International Space Station have seat restraints so that astronauts do not lift off the toilet seat because a fart released in weightlessness can act as a propulsive force.

The Fart Side: Blowing in the Wind!

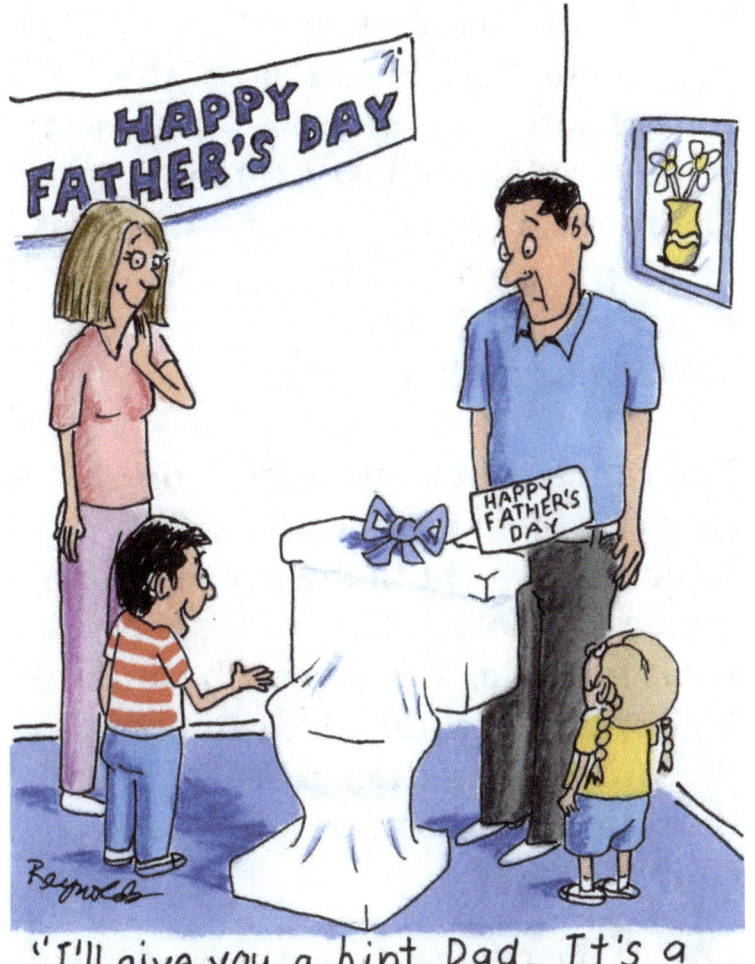

The Funny Side Collection

Ronald Wilson Reagan (1911 – 2004) was the fortieth President of the United Sates. An apocryphal story is related to Her Majesty, Queen Elizabeth II of Great Britain who was visiting the presidential ranch, Rancho Cielo, in the Santa Ynez Mountains of California.

The ranch is at a high elevation (Rancho Cielo is Spanish for Sky Ranch) and as both the president and queen are horse aficionados they went for a ride on the ranch trails. At higher altitude, the atmospheric pressure is less than at sea level and thus the volume of gasses expands (Boyle's Law).

The horse's intestinal tract likewise experienced expanding gasses, and

The Fart Side: Blowing in the Wind!

being natural animals they release it at will, even if they are in the presence of a Royal Queen and President. Along the trail the Queen's horse became increasingly flatulent, with noisy and pungent emissions.

The smell became overwhelming and unbearable, and the Queen felt obliged to apologize for her horse's gassiness by making the following comment to Mr. Reagan:

"Mr. President, I really must apologize for the terrible aroma."

Mr. Reagan politely responded, "Your Majesty, you needn't have apologized at all. In fact, if you hadn't said anything, I would have thought it was the horses!

The Funny Side Collection

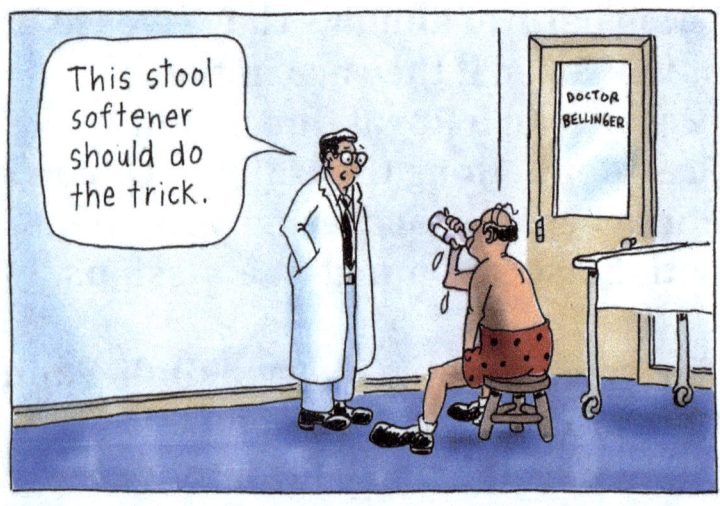

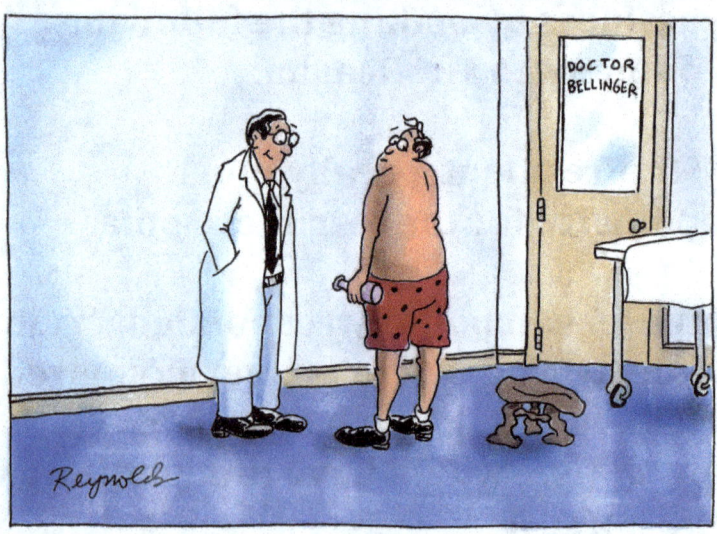

The Fart Side: Blowing in the Wind!

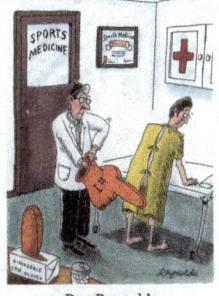

Dan Reynolds
Joseph Weiss, MD

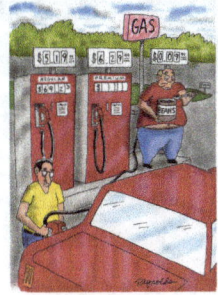

Dan Reynolds
Joseph Weiss, MD

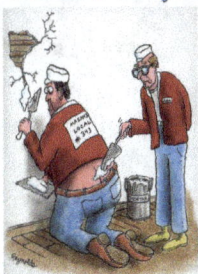

Dan Reynolds
Joseph Weiss, MD

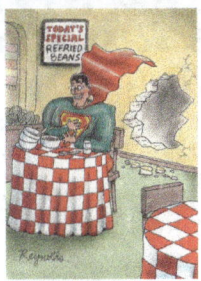

Dan Reynolds
Joseph Weiss, MD

Available in 5"x7" (96 pages) Pocket Rocket! and 6"x9" (122 pages) Expanded Full Blast! editions

www.thefunnysidecollection.com

The Funny Side Collection

Dan Reynolds

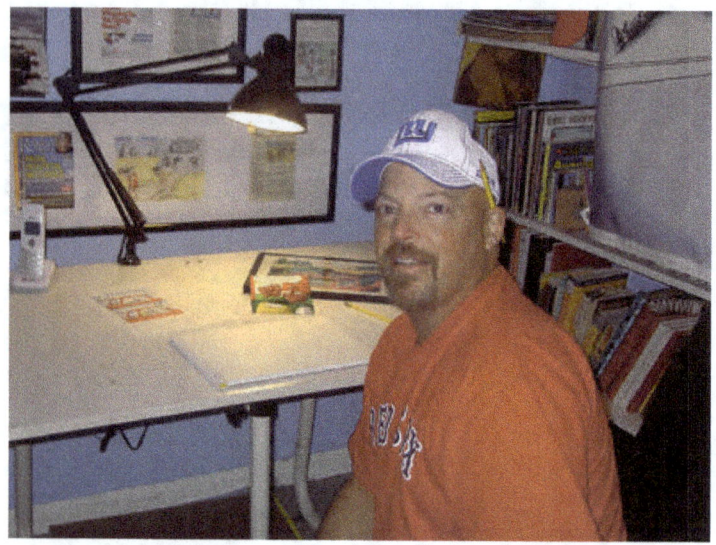

Dan Reynolds began drawing cartoons in December of 1989. He draws and eats left-handed. He plays ping pong and pool left-handed. He throws, kicks and bats right-handed. Like a box of chocolates, you never know what you're going to get, but you will like most of them and they'll keep you coming back. Unlike chocolates, REYNOLDS UNWRAPPED cartoons are not fattening.

Dan's cartoons are seen by millions of readers across the US, Canada and points beyond all the way down under in Australia. His work is seen in every issue of Reader's Digest (where he is known for his cow, pig, and chicken cartoons).

The Fart Side: Blowing in the Wind!

His cartoons have appeared on HBO's, The Sopranos, the cover of a National Lampoon cartoon book collection, and on greeting cards all throughout the United States. His work also appears in many other places as well.

Sign-up for Dan's daily REYNOLDS UNWRAPPED e-mail cartoon for only $12 for a whole year. E-mail Dan at reynoldsunwrapped@gmail.com for details. Dan's website is **www.reynoldsunwrapped.weebly.com**

The Fart Side series and other items are available at:
www.thefunnysidecollection.com

The Funny Side Collection

Joseph Weiss, M.D.

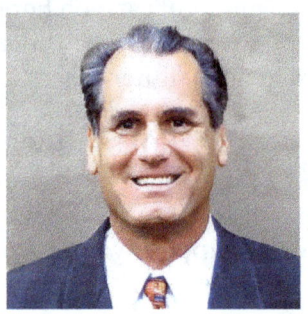

GI Joe is Clinical Professor of Medicine in the Division of Gastroenterology, Department of Medicine, at the University of California, San Diego. He is a Fellow of the American College of Physicians, Fellow of the American Gastroenterological Association, and a Senior Fellow of the American College of Gastroenterology. Dr. Weiss is the author of several dozen books on health, and is an accomplished professional speaker and humorist. His website is: **www.smartaskbooks.com**.

"Dr. Joseph Weiss' books provide an informative and entertaining approach to sharing insights about our digestive system and wellbeing." Deepak Chopra, MD

"Joseph Weiss, M.D. has a gift for books that are uniquely informative and entertaining. Jack Canfield Coauthor of the Chicken Soup for the Soul® series

The Fart Side series and other items are available at:
www.thefunnysidecollection.com

The Fart Side: Blowing in the Wind!

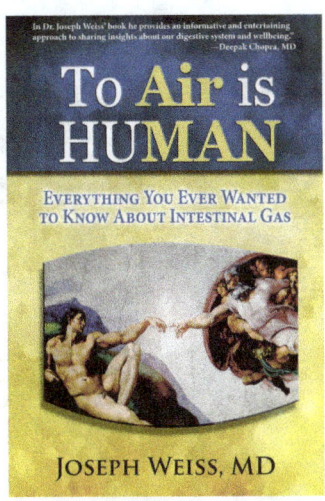

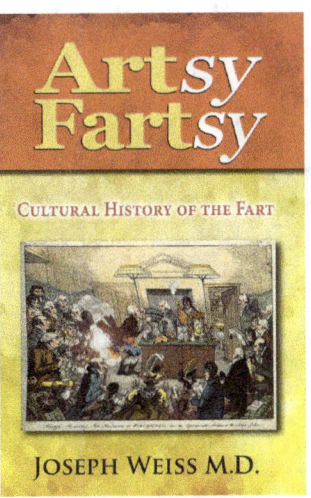

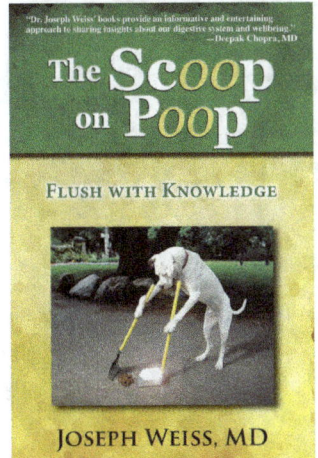

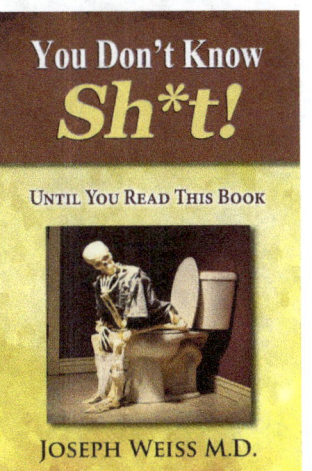

www.smartaskbooks.com

The Funny Side Collection

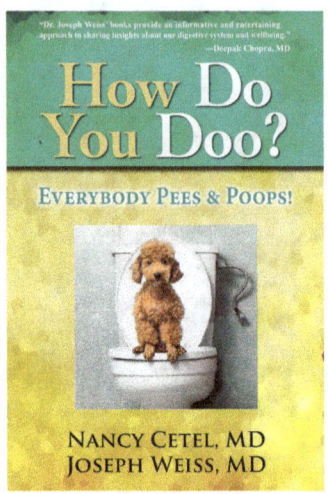
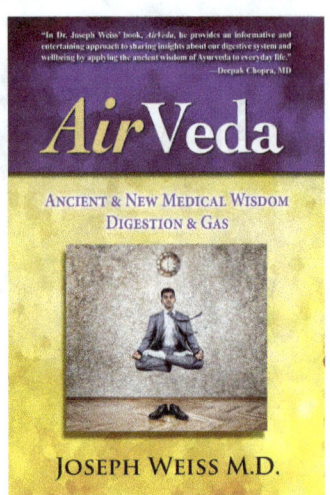
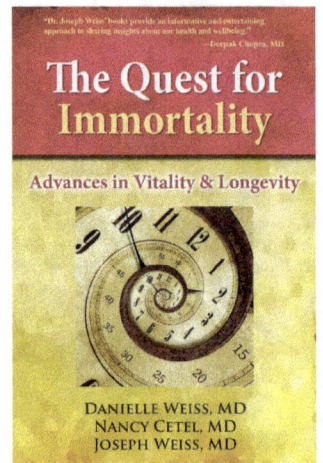
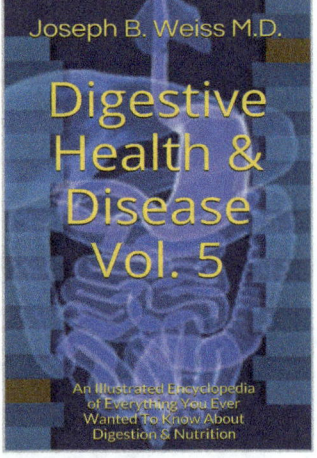

www.smartaskbooks.com

www.ingramcontent.com/pod-product-compliance
Lightning Source LLC
Chambersburg PA
CBHW071533080526
44588CB00011B/1659